Dr Gerald Coakley is a consult
gist specializing in post-viral
worked in the NHS for more th
London and Nottingham he was awarded an Arthritis Research
Campaign Fellowship, allowing him to conduct research in
immunology and immunogenetics relating to rheumatoid arthritis and Felty's syndrome at Guy's Hospital. In the NHS he has
a busy practice dealing with a wide variety of autoimmune and
inflammatory conditions, such as rheumatoid arthritis, lupus
and vasculitis. He was chair of the Education and Training
Committee at the British Society for Rheumatology from
2019 to 2022. Since 2001 he has been involved in the care of
people with ME/CFS and runs a private weekly fatigue clinic
at Keats House, London Bridge, and at the Harley Street Clinic.

Beverly Knops, Dip COT, MRCOT, is a Specialist Occupational Therapist with more than thirty years' experience. She
has spent the majority of her career working with people experiencing persistent pain and fatigue. She worked in North
Bristol NHS Trust (NBT) for twenty-nine years, starting in the
rheumatology service, then moving into the Specialist Pain and
ME/CFS services. Beverly says her main achievement at NBT
was developing and leading the patient volunteer programme.
She trained and supervised patients with lived experience who
are now involved in all aspects of the service, including co-
facilitating self-management courses. During this time she also
spent a period of nine years working one day a week for the
Bath Paediatric ME/CFS service, developing her knowledge
and expertise in this age group. In 2012 Beverly started work as
an associate therapist with Vitality360, a private company
working exclusively with people experiencing pain and fatigue.
In 2018 she was asked to take on the management of the company and, following a difficult decision in 2021 to leave the
NHS, she now leads this specialist team full-time. Beverly is a
trustee of the British Association of Clinicians working in
ME/CFS (BACME), where she actively contributes to the
training stream. She is passionate about sharing knowledge and
skills with other health professionals and has run numerous
training events throughout the country in person and online.

PENGUIN LIFE EXPERTS SERIES

The Penguin Life Experts series equips readers with simple but vital information on common health issues and empowers readers to get to know their own bodies to better improve their health. Books in the series include:

Managing Your Migraine
by Dr Katy Munro

* * * * *

Preparing for the Perimenopause and Menopause
by Dr Louise Newson

* * * * *

Keeping Your Heart Healthy
by Dr Boon Lim

* * * * *

Understanding Allergy
by Dr Sophie Farooque

* * * * *

Managing IBS
by Dr Lisa Das

* * * * *

Living with ME and Chronic Fatigue Syndrome
by Dr Gerald Coakley and Beverly Knops

Living with ME and Chronic Fatigue Syndrome

DR GERALD COAKLEY AND BEVERLY KNOPS

PENGUIN LIFE

AN IMPRINT OF

PENGUIN BOOKS

PENGUIN LIFE

UK | USA | Canada | Ireland | Australia
India | New Zealand | South Africa

Penguin Life is part of the Penguin Random House group of companies
whose addresses can be found at global.penguinrandomhouse.com.

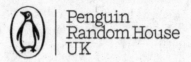

First published 2022
001

Copyright © Dr Gerald Coakley and Beverly Knops, 2022

The moral right of the authors has been asserted

Set in 12.5/14.75pt Garamond MT Std
Typeset by Jouve (UK), Milton Keynes
Printed and bound in Great Britain by Clays Ltd, Elcograf S.p.A.

The authorized representative in the EEA is Penguin Random House Ireland,
Morrison Chambers, 32 Nassau Street, Dublin D02 YH68

A CIP catalogue record for this book is available from the British Library

ISBN: 978-0-241-55721-1

www.greenpenguin.co.uk

To Luiz, my partner of three decades, for nourishing,
supporting and challenging me through thick and thin.
Dr Gerald Coakley

To my husband Simon, who has always believed in me.
When I say, 'I can't do it', he always says 'Yes, you can.'
Beverly Knops

Contents

Introduction   1

1 Classical ME/CFS   21
2 PVFS and Other Fatigue-Related
   Syndromes   42
3 Theories Regarding Causation   65
4 Self-Management Strategies   89
5 Treatment Options: Medications
   and Supplements   109
6 Nutrition and Food   126
7 ME/CFS, Work and Education   141
8 How Best to Support a Loved One
   with ME/CFS   158
9 Questions to Ask Your Healthcare
   Professional   168
10 Referral to Specialist Services   175
11 Life after ME/CFS   189

CONTENTS

Conclusion: Living with ME/CFS   205

Notes   209

Further Reading and Resources   223

Acknowledgements   229

Introduction

Fatigue is a very common symptom, which we all experience at times. But in its more severe and persistent forms it is difficult to define and to explain, both for people with fatigue and for their doctors. No medical student goes to university to become a fatigue doctor, because this is a speciality that does not, at least yet, exist.

I (Gerald) first became curious about chronic fatigue syndrome, as it was then termed, around twenty years ago, shortly after I was appointed as a consultant rheumatologist in London and started to see patients privately. Most of the patients I saw were like those in my National Health Service (NHS) practice, which – because I was a rheumatologist – meant people with suspected inflammatory conditions such as rheumatoid arthritis or psoriatic arthritis, inflammatory spinal diseases like ankylosing spondylitis, autoimmune disorders such as lupus, or metabolic conditions like gout. But I was referred some private patients who had been receiving unorthodox treatments for what we now know as myalgic encephalomyelitis/chronic fatigue syndrome (ME/CFS) and whose usual treating physicians had either retired or died.

The first patients I saw had been receiving something known as a Myers' cocktail given intravenously on a regular basis for many years, and I was asked whether I would be prepared to continue prescribing this cocktail. Knowing nothing about it, I looked it up. It turns out that it was invented in the 1960s by Dr John Myers of Baltimore, Maryland, and has been used by complementary medical practitioners to treat a wide range of conditions, including ME/CFS, asthma, migraine, fibromyalgia (see page 53) and chronic sinusitis, among others. It is a bright-yellow liquid given by infusion, containing a blend of B vitamins, including thiamine, niacinamide, pyridoxine and hydroxocobalamin (vitamin B_{12}), as well as vitamin D, magnesium and calcium.

Intrigued, I looked for evidence that this treatment was effective in ME/CFS. I have a PhD in molecular immuno-genetics, and at the time was chairing a national guideline group seeking to define the optimal treatment for septic arthritis (a life-threatening bacterial joint infection), so I was very familiar with the world of evidence-based medicine grounded in systematic reviews of the scientific literature. When I looked into Myers' infusions, it turned out that while many people with ME/CFS report taking vitamin supplements and believe they are helpful, there was absolutely no clinical-trial evidence to suggest Myers' infusions are in any way effective in treating ME/CFS. Indeed, since then multiple published systematic reviews have concluded that vitamins are no better than placebos in ME/CFS unless the patient has a proven vitamin deficiency, and there are in fact no approved treatments specific to ME/CFS.[1] I was happy to see the patients, but not to offer them a treatment that I was convinced was ineffective and not without risk.

I drew several conclusions from these early encounters. First, the absence of any effective treatment for a condition as potentially disabling as ME/CFS does not reflect well on the current state of medical research and practice. Second, when conventional medicine has nothing to offer, people with disabling conditions like ME/CFS will quite rightly not give up trying to improve their health, but will look to alternative and fringe medicine to find support. When they do that, they are, unfortunately, at the mercy of people who are credulous, ill informed or, worse still, simply want to exploit their vulnerability for financial gain. I have met patients who have spent thousands of pounds on quack treatments such as ozone therapy, or on fake diagnostics such as the Vega machine (an electroacupuncture device developed in the 1970s, which has been shown in numerous studies to be useless). Third, some doctors in the private sector appear to be in on this potentially lucrative trade, which I can only regard as disreputable. It was not a path I wanted to follow myself. Incidentally, today Myers' infusions are beloved by some celebrities and people with more money than sense to help them recover from hangovers, to prevent wrinkles or as a general pick-me-up. There are even companies that market Myers' cocktail as a way to keep your immune system healthy, for 'reinvigoration' and to 'transform your health', at a cost of £250 per infusion.

Realizing there was a sizeable group of people with ME/CFS who were receiving little or no help from the NHS and were seeking answers in the private sector, I wanted to try to do something to help, based on the best up-to-date evidence, rather than simply providing a service for which there was a demand. So it was that – simultaneously with the launch of guidelines in 2007 by the UK National Institute for Health and Care Excellence (NICE), which recommended cognitive behavioural therapy and graded activity as the only effective treatments for ME/CFS – I set up the Fatigue Clinic in London working with a multidisciplinary team, aimed at offering such treatment to those who wanted it.

Since that time, the 2007 NICE guidelines and the treatments they supported have faced a deluge of criticism, some of it deserved, some not, in my opinion (we will be looking at treatment options in more detail later in the book). Revised NICE guidelines were released in 2021, which were clear in stating that the currently available treatments are not curative, while also not offering any new or alternative treatments in place of the previously recommended ones. Some in the ME/CFS community see this revision as a huge step forward, because they believe it will unleash a tidal wave of biomedical research that will quickly lead to effective new treatments. Others question whether jettisoning approaches that can help many people but do not help all – when there is no guarantee that any effective novel treatment will emerge for the foreseeable future – really represents progress.

What is not in doubt is that people with ME/CFS benefit from well-intentioned clinicians experienced in helping people with the condition, from being believed and feeling understood, and from getting useful practical advice on how to manage their fatigue and its impact on their work or studies and on their personal and social lives. Irrespective of all the controversies that surround ME/CFS and its treatment, I find it professionally rewarding to see people living successfully with the condition. I feel I have learned as much from them as I hope they have from my experience of trying to help people with this sometimes very challenging condition.

Why we wrote this book, by Beverly Knops

When Gerald first asked me to co-author this book, I felt fearful. Not fearful that I couldn't do it or had nothing to say, but fearful of attracting attention. This is a common feeling among clinicians in this clinical area.

Over the next few days I realized this could be a great opportunity for me to contribute to the narrative around ME/CFS and offer some well-thought-through practical advice to a wider audience than those patients I personally see in my work.

I have worked as an occupational therapist with people experiencing symptoms of ME/CFS for more than fifteen years. During this time I have seen hundreds of people, read extensively, attended conferences and training events, led training courses, learned from my colleagues and, most importantly, learned from each and every person I have worked with.

I base my therapeutic work on the best evidence, which I extract from all these sources. Each programme is different, founded on the values and goals of the individual within the context of their lives, but I hope that I have extracted here some common themes that readers can apply to their own lives. I have attempted to include throughout my writing the voices of many of those I have worked with: their voices need to be heard, and so does mine.

How to use this book

As clinicians and authors, we have put the reader at the centre of this book and have designed it with *you* in mind. The book is not meant to be read in one sitting; you can dip in and out and read it at your own pace. Nor do you have to read it from cover to cover: if you find it more useful, filter out those chapters that are not relevant to you – for example, advice on education, if you have long left school; or advice on the workplace, if you are self-employed.

We have taken care with the structure, so that it is as concise and practical as possible. Of course ME/CFS will affect people differently, from being relatively minor to completely overwhelming, so we have based a lot of the practical advice on those who are moderately affected.

What is ME/CFS?

Fatigue is a common, non-specific symptom with many causes, including physical health problems, medication or other substance use and psychological conditions, including anxiety, depression and 'burnout' or work-related stress (see the table below).

Medical conditions associated with fatigue

System	Condition
Cardiac	Heart failure
Respiratory	Obstructive sleep apnoea, chronic obstructive pulmonary disease
Endocrine/metabolic	Thyroid disease, adrenal insufficiency, chronic kidney or liver disease, coeliac disease
Haematological	Anaemia, cancer
Rheumatological	Rheumatoid arthritis, lupus, Sjögren's syndrome, inflammatory muscle disease
Neurological	Multiple sclerosis
Medication	Benzodiazepines, antidepressants, beta-blockers, opiates, gabapentin, pregabalin
Substance use	Alcohol, opiates, cocaine, cannabis
Psychological	Anxiety, depression, burnout

The term 'fatigue' is used by different people to mean different things. It can reflect a difficulty in initiating activity, due to a subjective sense of weakness, or a reduced capacity to maintain activity; while for others it refers to mental fatigue – difficulty with concentration or memory. Often there is a combination of these symptoms, and up to one-third of primary-care consultations are about feeling tired all the time.[2] In many cases, fatigue is either short-lived or not intrusive, but when it persists for more than a few months in the absence of a clear cause and interferes with normal daily activities, the possibility of ME/CFS has to be considered.

There are several definitions of ME/CFS currently in common use, and the terms ME, CFS and ME/CFS or CFS/ME are often used interchangeably. Doctors tend not to favour the term 'myalgic encephalomyelitis' – which literally translates as 'brain inflammation with aching muscles' – because there is little evidence of brain or muscle inflammation in the condition (see page 17 for further information). ME/CFS is characterized by the onset, either abrupt or gradual, of persistent disabling fatigue, together with unrefreshing sleep, problems with cognition (such as memory, thinking and concentration), muscle and joint aches, headaches and tender lymph nodes without enlargement, lasting for more than a few months.

A hallmark of the condition, which is essential to the diagnosis and differentiates it from other commoner forms of fatigue, is known as post-exertional malaise

(PEM). This represents a group of symptoms (fatigue, headaches, muscle aches, insomnia or thinking problems) that increase following mental or physical exertion, lasting twenty-four hours or more. It is this symptom that often limits people with ME/CFS to only a few hours per day of productive activity, with the remainder of the day spent resting.

The World Health Organization classifies ME/CFS as a neurological illness, although the majority of neurologists do not share that view.[3] However it is classified, ME/CFS can cause profound, prolonged illness and disability, which has a substantial impact on people with the condition and on their carers. The many uncertainties about the causes, diagnosis and best management serve only to worsen its impact.

How prevalent is ME/CFS?

The Medical Research Council estimates that ME/CFS affects 250,000 people in the UK, which is to say roughly three in every 1,000 people. In the US it is estimated that up to 2.5 million people, from teenage years to middle age – of all ethnicities and socioeconomic backgrounds – are affected.[4] The condition is three times more common in women than in men[5] for reasons that are unclear, but similar ratios are seen in, for example, rheumatoid arthritis, systemic lupus erythematosus and multiple sclerosis. ME/CFS typically first affects people from their adolescence until the age of around fifty.[6]

How is ME/CFS defined?

There are several definitions in common use, and none are universally accepted. In common with most illness classification criteria, the main concern of the scientists who created those criteria was to tightly define a uniform patient population for research studies rather than to create a tool for use in the consulting room. There must be a degree of pragmatism in applying these criteria to people who are attending their physicians for routine clinical care rather than for entry into a research study. For this reason, we favour the pragmatic definition used by NICE in the 2021 guideline.[7] They advised clinicians to consider ME/CFS when an individual presents with fatigue showing all of the following features:

- **Debilitating fatigue** that is worsened by activity, is not caused by excessive cognitive, physical, emotional or social exertion and is not significantly relieved by rest.

- **Post-exertional malaise after activity**, in which the onset of worsening of symptoms is often delayed by hours or days, is disproportionate to the activity and has a prolonged recovery time that may last hours, days, weeks or longer.

- **Unrefreshing sleep or sleep disturbance** (or both), which may include feeling exhausted, feeling flu-like and stiff on waking, broken or shallow sleep, altered sleep patterns or excessive daytime sleepiness, known as hypersomnia.

- **Cognitive difficulties** (sometimes described as 'brain fog'), which may include problems in finding words or numbers, difficulty in speaking, slowed responsiveness, short-term memory problems and difficulty concentrating or multitasking.

NICE advised that a diagnosis of ME/CFS should be suspected in the presence of all these symptoms after other possible diagnoses have been excluded, where the person's ability to engage in occupational, educational, social or personal activities is significantly reduced from pre-illness levels and the symptoms have persisted for at least six weeks in an adult, or four weeks in a child or young person.

Alternative criteria

There are numerous alternative diagnostic and classification criteria, including the 1994 US Centers for Disease Control ('Fukuda') Criteria, and the 2003 Canadian Consensus Criteria (which made the feature of post-exertional malaise pre-eminent). There are also the 2010 Canadian Consensus Criteria, the 2011 International Consensus Criteria, and the 2015 US National Academy of Medicine criteria. The 1991 Oxford criteria have largely fallen out of favour as they do not include PEM, so there is concern that these criteria capture individuals with non-specific fatigue, or fatigue associated with anxiety and depression, and therefore could over-state the benefits of psychological therapies in ME/CFS. Full consideration of the various criteria lies beyond the scope of this book, but for those who would like to learn more, there is a thorough exploration in a paper from the Mayo Foundation for Medical Education and Research.[8]

Mild, moderate and severe ME/CFS: what are the differences?

A common problem that we come across in our everyday clinical practice is that the condition is highly variable, with some individuals being able to live a more or less normal life, and others being housebound or bedbound. This means that some people who have ME/CFS at the milder end of the spectrum either do not believe their diagnosis is correct or have difficulty being believed by others, who know only of the most severely affected group. Again, this is where the 2021 NICE guidelines are helpful, because they grade severity thus:

- **Mild ME/CFS**: People with mild ME/CFS are mobile, can care for themselves and can do light domestic tasks (sometimes needing support), but may have difficulties with mobility. Most are still working or in education, but to do this they have probably stopped all leisure and social pursuits. They often have reduced hours, take days off and use the weekend to cope with the remainder of the week.

- **Moderate ME/CFS**: People with moderate ME/CFS have reduced mobility and are restricted in all activities of daily living, although they may have peaks and troughs in their level of symptoms and their ability to do activities. They have usually stopped work or education and need rest periods, often in the afternoon for one or two hours. Their sleep at night is generally of poor quality and disturbed.

- **Severe ME/CFS**: People with severe ME/CFS are unable to do any activity for themselves or can carry out minimal daily tasks only (such as face-washing and cleaning their teeth). They have severe cognitive difficulties and depend on a wheelchair for mobility. They are often unable to leave the house or have a severe and prolonged after-effect if they do so. They may also spend most of their time in bed and are often extremely sensitive to light and noise.

- **Very severe ME/CFS**: People with very severe ME/CFS are in bed all day and are dependent on care. They need help with personal hygiene and eating and are highly sensitive to sensory stimuli. Some people may not be able to swallow and may need to be tube-fed.

This wide range of symptoms and severity may go some way towards explaining why living with ME/CFS can be so distressing. Medical science still cannot explain why some people get this condition, and there is no very effective treatment. While many people with ME/CFS are able to live a fairly normal life despite their symptoms, a significant minority – in our experience, perhaps a quarter – have symptoms so severe that they are confined to their house or even their bed. In the worst cases, people are unable to feed or toilet themselves.

Worryingly, studies show that suicide rates among ME/CFS sufferers are well above the national average. In a 2016 analysis of the medical records of 2,000 people diagnosed with ME/CFS in England and Wales,[9] it was found that the rate of death by suicide was six times higher in people with ME/CFS than in the general population. In the US a recent review found that compared with the national average of 4 per cent of the population who had contemplated suicide, the rate among those moderately to severely affected by ME/CFS was between 40 and 60 per cent.[10]

An important part of the challenge of ME/CFS is that many people with the condition are faced with prejudice and disbelief, both from wider society and, at times, within the medical profession. They can feel stigmatized by those who do not understand their illness, and as a result they may have lost trust in health and other caring services. It is our experience that acknowledging the reality of living with ME/CFS is vital in gaining the trust of the patients we see, and it takes time to build supportive and empathic relationships. Sadly, we do not always succeed.

As professionals, we are mindful that private healthcare is expensive and that not everyone is in a position to access it. Even if they were, provision of specialist services is patchy in the UK in both the NHS and the private sector, and this is also the experience of many people with ME/CFS worldwide. That is why, through this book, we wish to address a real need for people who have recently developed ME/CFS to access sensible, evidence-based information. You will find accessible information here about the nature of the condition, how it may progress over time and what you can do to help improve your health. We also offer practical advice on the key questions to ask your health professional; how to handle areas such as school or university attendance; employment issues, including a return to work; and, where symptoms are severe and unresponsive to treatment, how to access financial support.

ME/CFS affects people differently and there is no one-size-fits-all approach, but we both see the real value of hearing the stories of those who are living with the condition, so this book also contains first-hand accounts from people sharing their stories about living with ME/CFS. Whether you have recently developed ME/CFS or a loved one has, we hope this book will inform, provide much-needed support and empower you.

> **What's in a name: the complicated history of**
> **the term 'myalgic encephalomyelitis'**
> **The term 'myalgic encephalomyelitis' (ME)**
> **was first coined in 1955 by a physician from**
> **Iceland called Björn Sigurdsson. He**
> **suggested the name 'benign myalgic**
> **encephalomyelitis' after noting similarities**

between two outbreaks of illness among staff at London's Royal Free Hospital in 1955 and an earlier outbreak in Akureyi, Iceland, in 1949.

Patients in both outbreaks had symptoms including muscle pain, vertigo and a low-grade fever. However, Sigurdsson noted some similarities in abnormalities in the cerebrospinal fluid – a clear, colourless liquid found in the brain and spinal cord that helps protect against sudden impact or injury and assists the central nervous system to function properly – in patients from both outbreaks. Specifically, he found slightly raised cerebrospinal fluid white-cell counts and protein levels in four of eight cases.

Sigurdsson described symptoms and signs of damage to the brain and spinal cord, along with protracted muscle pain, that led him to coin the term, which means muscle pain (myalgia) related to central-nervous-system inflammation (encephalomyelitis).

Fast-forward sixty years and 'ME' is the term preferred by many patient associations, which feel that the term 'chronic fatigue syndrome' is either dismissive of the severity of their complaints or risks inclusion within the ME/CFS diagnostic category of people who have non-specific fatigue or fatigue due to mental-health problems, and could therefore under-play the illness severity of those with ME.

For many physicians, however, the term ME is problematic. Traditionally inflammation of any tissue – the brain included – is confirmed by microscopic examination of that tissue. Clearly, sampling brain tissue is hazardous and extremely invasive, so it is seldom done except in the diagnosis of brain tumours. Therefore for years we have relied on post-mortem examinations of people with ME/CFS. A few post-mortem studies have been reported, and a variety of abnormalities found, including several with inflammation in the dorsal-root ganglia of their spinal cords (this is a cluster of cells that helps transmit sensory messages of pain and touch) and some with degenerative changes in their brain. None had classical signs of inflammatory brain disease. A number of ME associations are encouraging members to sign up for post-mortem brain studies, but these are difficult to arrange, and in our opinion it is unlikely that a significant breakthrough in understanding will come from such approaches.

Another way to look at the question of brain inflammation is through modern imaging techniques. These include positron emission tomography (PET) scanning, which creates a 3D image in which substances bound to positron-emitting isotopes are introduced into the body, allowing radiologists to identify which brain regions are activated in real time, and magnetic resonance spectroscopy (MRS), which looks for biochemical changes in the brain.

In 2014 Japanese scientists reported neuroinflammation in patients with ME/CFS by PET scanning.[11] They found increased PET signal in the midbrain of patients with ME/CFS. However, this study has not been replicated and there are complex methodological issues, which mean it is not yet established or widely accepted that these findings are valid.

There are arguments that MRS is a more reliable way to detect inflammation. There have been several studies of the brains of people with ME/CFS using MRS, some of which have shown increased brain lactate levels. However, no study has found increased lactate in the same brain region, which again raises concerns about the accuracy and validity of the measurement.

The variation in research findings is thought to reflect a wide variety of experimental designs, diagnostic criteria, subject populations, comparison control groups, brain regions examined and metabolites targeted.

The neuroimaging data in ME/CFS were recently reviewed by a team of academics working in neurotherapeutics at Harvard Medical School.[12] They surmised that:

The ME/CFS research field has been stuck in a somewhat defensive posture, with a focus on demonstrating 'this is a real condition' by showing significant biological differences between patients and controls. We believe this has led to a situation in which too much is made of the specifics reported by descriptive studies, and not enough emphasis has been placed on potential mechanisms driving symptoms.

They went on to suggest a greater focus on research methods and a concentration not only on whether there are differences between patients and controls, but rather on whether a significant result can inform our understanding of disease mechanisms.

The team asserts (and we agree) that the relationship of ME/CFS to neuroinflammation is a fundamental question, not yet resolved, that needs to be addressed from multiple research angles. It must take into account that ME/CFS causes changes to lifestyles that could explain some of the study results (such as sedentary lifestyles or dietary alterations).

In our opinion, the jury remains out on whether or not (despite the name) there is in fact an inflammatory brain disease that results in the condition we know as ME/CFS. At present we believe that neuroinflammation in ME/CFS is an interesting hypothesis: no more, no less.

1. Classical ME/CFS

Anyone can get ME/CFS at any point during their life, but the peak age of onset is between the early teens and the age of fifty. It affects men albeit less commonly than women, irrespective of social class or occupation. The cause is unknown, although various suggestions have been made, including viral infection, autoimmunity, neurological disorders and psychological distress. Most clinicians working in this area would recognize that ME/CFS is probably not a single condition, but rather a set of symptoms that can result from a variety of different causes or processes. While anybody can be affected by ME/CFS, there are common patterns in many of those who present with symptoms fulfilling the criteria for the condition.

In this chapter we look at the predisposing factors (those that put a person at risk of developing a condition, such as genetics) and at precipitating factors (such as a specific event or trigger) for ME/CFS.

Predisposing factors

While nobody is immune from the risk of developing ME/CFS, there are common factors in many people presenting with new onset of fatigue symptoms that go on to fulfil criteria for ME/CFS. It is associated with a variety of other conditions that are currently not well understood or easily explained, including fibromyalgia (see page 53), irritable bowel syndrome, chronic headache, chronic pelvic pain and joint hypermobility. People with a prior history of any of these diagnoses are considered to have an increased vulnerability to developing ME/CFS (we will be covering this in more detail in the next chapter).

A family history of anxiety is associated with a three-fold increased risk of developing the condition.[1] It is likely that genetic factors are involved, and there is a higher prevalence of ME/CFS among family members, particularly twins.[2]

There is also a role for stress in both predisposing and probably also precipitating ME/CFS.[3] One Swedish study, which examined 41,000 twins over a twenty-five-year period, demonstrated that after accounting for genetic factors, self-reported stress was associated with an almost sixfold increased risk of developing an ME/CFS-like illness.[4]

While the triggering event for ME/CFS is very often a viral infection, such as a cold or flu, humans have coexisted with these viruses for millennia, and most adults will experience a least two viral upper-respiratory-tract infections per year without developing ME/CFS, including those who later go on to develop the condition. So to make sense of why someone with new-onset ME/CFS has developed the condition after a viral infection this year, rather than last year or five years ago, we explore the possible stressors in the months prior to the onset that might have contributed to an increased vulnerability.

Common stressors

Common stressors that we see in our patients are academic exams and major life events such as the illness or death of a loved one, a house move or renovations, stressful work environments and dysfunctional family relationships. Naturally, most of the people with ME/CFS that we see, in whom academic examinations could be relevant, are adolescents and young adults, most of whom will experience persistent stress over many months in the run-up to their end-of-school examinations or at university. Indeed we see many first-year university students with ME/CFS, probably due to the combination of several stressful life events (such as relocating, separation from parents for the first time, a new academic environment and multiple examinations) with repeated exposure to fellow students, who represent a perfect breeding ground for viruses such as Epstein–Barr, the virus that causes glandular fever. One recent study of 4,500 US university students found that 238 (just over 5 per cent) contracted glandular fever. The study authors found that fifty-five (23 per cent) of those students with glandular fever went on to meet the criteria for ME/CFS six months later.[5]

The precise mechanisms by which persistent stress increases the vulnerability to develop ME/CFS are not clear. However, it is known that stress can affect the body's delicate systems for regulating its hormones and adrenaline levels in response to internal challenges (such as infections and injuries) or environmental challenges (the fight-or-flight response).

The body's stress-response system involves two parts of the brain: the hypothalamus, a small area near the base of the brain, and the pituitary gland, a small pea-sized gland. It also involves the adrenal glands, which are situated above the kidneys in the abdomen. Collectively these are known as the hypothalamic/pituitary/adrenal (HPA) axis.

Stress stimulates the hypothalamus to release a hormone called corticotropin-releasing hormone (CRH), which in turn stimulates the pituitary gland to release a second hormone called adrenocorticotropic hormone (ACTH). This travels through the bloodstream to the adrenal-gland cortex (the outer part of the gland), where the release of the hormone cortisol happens within hours. In parallel, the hypothalamus can directly and immediately stimulate the core of the adrenal gland (the medulla) to release adrenaline through the autonomic nervous system – a network of cells that regulates and supports many different internal processes without our being conscious of it.

In an acutely stressful situation, such as the need to fight or run from danger, these changes are helpful. However, persistent stress has many adverse effects on the immune system. ACTH and cortisol suppress the immune system and block various protective responses.[6] Therefore down-regulating the immune system is one of the effects of elevated cortisol levels, and this is thought to be one mechanism by which persistent or chronic stress can increase vulnerability to infections – or to those infections having more severe consequences than they would otherwise have. A diagram summarizing these complex interactions is shown opposite.

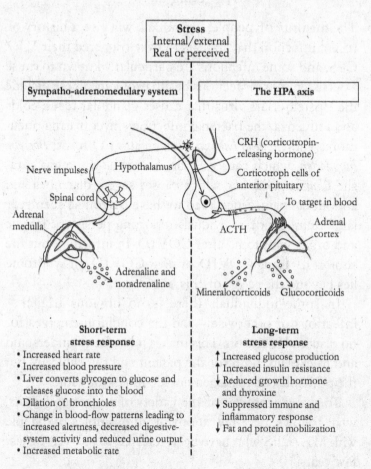

Stress
Internal/external
Real or perceived

Sympatho-adrenomedulary system

The HPA axis

CRH (corticotropin-releasing hormone)

Corticotroph cells of anterior pituitary

Nerve impulses   Hypothalamus

Spinal cord

To target in blood

Adrenal medulla

ACTH

Adrenal cortex

Adrenaline and noradrenaline

Mineralocorticoids   Glucocorticoids

Short-term stress response
- Increased heart rate
- Increased blood pressure
- Liver converts glycogen to glucose and releases glucose into the blood
- Dilation of bronchioles
- Change in blood-flow patterns leading to increased alertness, decreased digestive-system activity and reduced urine output
- Increased metabolic rate

Long-term stress response
↑ Increased glucose production
↑ Increased insulin resistance
↓ Reduced growth hormone and thyroxine
↓ Suppressed immune and inflammatory response
↓ Fat and protein mobilization

The stress response system: stress signals affect the hypothalamus in the brain, which through the nervous system triggers the adrenal medulla to immediately release adrenaline and noradrenaline (the fight-or-flight response). More slowly, the hypothalamus also releases hormones within the HPA axis that influence the release of the stress hormone cortisol and other hormones from the adrenal cortex.

The stress response system

Triggering factors

The majority of people, but not all, will give a history of recent infection that appears to have triggered their ME/CFS, and some infections are particularly known to cause a persistent post-infectious health problem. These include the Epstein–Barr virus that causes glandular fever; colds and influenza, the bacterial infections mycoplasma pneumonia and *Coxiella burnetii*, which causes Q fever; *Borrelia burgdorferi*, which causes Lyme disease; and the gut parasite *Giardia duodenalis*, which causes severe diarrhoea and abdominal pain. Since 2020 we have of course seen very large numbers of individuals reporting persistent fatigue and other symptoms after COVID-19 infection, but the subject of Long COVID or post-COVID-19 syndrome lies beyond the scope of this book.

In some individuals there is no obvious trigger – infectious or otherwise – and the condition emerges for no discernible reason. This makes it harder to understand and to explain, both for the patient and the clinician, but the principles of management are much the same.

To give you an idea of the variety of triggering factors, what follows are a few anonymized examples of people with ME/CFS who have been referred to us over the last few years.

Steven, 33

Steven was on a sabbatical from his job working in finance in the City of London. He travelled extensively over several continents, clocking up 5,600km (3,500 miles) of cycling, and was also a regular gym-goer who had participated in several half-marathons.

When Steven returned to work he was keen to pay back his employers for granting him the sabbatical. He worked very long hours, but even so continued with a vigorous exercise regime in the gym. Two months after his return he noticed that the racing heart he expected to have during exercise was persisting for longer than it should after he stopped. Although he thought it was a little strange, he was not too worried.

Then, after a 160-km (100-mile) cycling trip, he woke up with chest pain and exhaustion. He saw a physician, had extensive tests, which were normal, and was thought to have suffered a viral chest infection with post-viral fatigue. Steven was advised to stop vigorous exercise, but unfortunately when he started gentle exercise four months later, he suffered post-exertional malaise that fulfilled the criteria for ME/CFS.

He had to take some sick days off work. He tried to get back to the gym, but even thirty minutes there would result in severe worsening of his fatigue for five days. He had the need to urinate more frequently and with greater urgency, and would feel feverish, although his temperature was always normal when he took it.

Extensive blood and cardiology testing came back with normal results. He was managing to continue at work with just the odd day off, but was no longer able to exercise or socialize. Unsurprisingly, in these circumstances, he was beginning to feel low in mood and sought help with understanding his symptoms and developing a plan for recovery. At the time of writing, Steve is still receiving support to help him find a more appropriate work–life balance, in part through a temporary reduction in work hours, and manage his symptoms effectively.

Nish, 32

Qualified accountant Nish suffered an episode of work stress so severe that he developed anxiety and depression. He had to take some time off work and was prescribed a course of antidepressants, which helped.

Nish returned to work, but the next year he caught glandular fever. He suffered from post-viral symptoms for many months, and although he was able to continue at work, he could only do so by stopping all socializing and exercise (which was hard for someone who used to cycle six days a week and go to the gym regularly). He spent almost all his time either working or sleeping.

He managed to sustain this pattern for four years before deciding that he needed some time out to concentrate on his health. He did some volunteer work and travelled extensively. While trekking in Africa he suffered a severe setback in his fatigue and malaise, from which he had not recovered at the time he went to a fatigue specialist three years later.

In fact Nish suffered a progressive deterioration. First he became unable to maintain his flat and moved back in with his parents. Then he stopped being able to cook, and finally lost even the ability to walk around his parents' garden. He became bedbound, and lost weight because eating was too tiring. He became increasingly withdrawn, immobile and depressed, and suffered daily thoughts of suicide. He spent a few days as a voluntary in-patient in a psychiatric unit.

After he was discharged, he spent all his time in a hospital bed that had been set up in his parents' living room. He had poor-quality, non-restorative sleep. He spent almost twenty-four hours a day horizontal and could only read for up to four minutes. He passed all his waking time either resting or listening to podcasts. We will be revisiting Nish's case in more detail in Chapter 3 (see page 82).

Katie, 19

Katie, a university student, presented with a long history of fatigue. This had started at the age of eleven, when she was thought to have contracted glandular fever. She had to take a lot of time off school because of her fatigue. Investigations including antibody testing, and an intestinal (duodenal) biopsy showed that she also had coeliac disease, which is known to be a cause of fatigue. She excluded gluten from her diet, and a repeat biopsy showed her gut mucosa had returned to normal. Unfortunately this did not help her fatigue problem, but she managed to complete her schooling and got good exam results, winning a place at university.

As well as marked fatigue, Katie also complained of sore throats, headaches and aching joints and muscles. She was known to have joint hypermobility (flexible joints that can be associated with joint pain). She was sleeping for ten hours a night, and for three hours during the day. Due to her fatigue, Katie could not exercise and suffered from post-exertional malaise for several days if she tried to. She could manage the ten-minute walk to university each day, but had taken six weeks off from her first year at university, due to her fatigue.

Her mood had been adversely affected, and she worried about her future and would at times be tearful and upset. She had several courses of counselling and talking therapy, without benefit. With the support of a therapist, Katie came to understand that while rest during an acute infection is appropriate, in the long term sleeping for thirteen hours in every twenty-four results in low-quality, non-restorative sleep. With difficulty, she managed to reduce this over a period of weeks to an eight-hour sleep habit. While fatigue symptoms remained, she was then able to complete her degree and move into the world of employment successfully.

What are the common signs and symptoms of ME/CFS?

Reaching a diagnosis of ME/CFS requires the presence of new-onset physical and mental fatigue symptoms for more than a few weeks, sufficient to result in a substantial reduction in usual levels of activity. That can include physical exercise, socializing, work or study, or a combination of any of these. It is a requirement of the diagnosis that the patient gives a history of post-exertional malaise, typically occurring twenty-four hours or more after unaccustomed physical, mental or social exertion. Apart from fatigue, other common and prominent symptoms in those with ME/CFS include:

- **Chronic musculoskeletal pain** in the absence of inflammation

- **Headache** with light and sound sensitivity

- **Cognitive dysfunction**, such as problems with concentration, thinking, memory and word-finding (these features are often termed 'brain fog', although this is a lay term without any precise medical meaning)

- **Sleep alteration**, which is almost universal in ME/CFS and can include insomnia or its opposite, hypersomnia: sleeping for anything up to twenty hours a day

- **Orthostatic intolerance**, described by many people – especially those who are mostly bedbound with severe ME/CFS – as dizziness when they stand, light-headedness, unsteadiness, nausea or vertigo with a fear of falling, or indeed fainting; these symptoms are relieved by lying down

- **Anxiety or depression**, and perhaps not surprisingly and as with any long-term health condition, around 40 per cent of people with ME/CFS suffer from depression or anxiety.[7] [8] While the majority of people with ME/CFS do not suffer from mental illness, it is important to screen for anxiety and depression, because if they are present they make the situation worse and are relatively easy to treat.

Investigations to reach a diagnosis

There are so many disorders that may result in fatigue that it can be difficult to know when to stop investigating. Understandably, many people diagnosed with or suspected of having ME/CFS find it frustrating to be told that the results of their investigations are all normal or negative, and want more tests to find some hidden or obscure condition. The role of the physician is to help navigate a sensible path between over-investigating, on the one hand, and missing potentially treatable pathologies that could reverse the fatigue problem, on the other.

I (Gerald) find that people often want lots of tests, but there is a balance to be struck. When results come back negative, that is reassuring for the doctor, but very often not for the patient. When results come back showing an abnormality, the patient will very often latch on to that as the cause of the fatigue, irrespective of whether or not that is biologically plausible. Most blood tests are designed to show a normal range that incorporates 95 per cent of the healthy population. This means that even among healthy individuals, 5 per cent of test results (or one in twenty) will be abnormal. The more tests one requests, the more results outside the normal range will be found, even in people of perfect health. But those abnormal results – even if irrelevant to the symptom of fatigue – will in themselves become a source of concern, prompting further tests to evaluate the abnormalities.

It is not uncommon in fatigue clinics to see patients

who have consulted multiple doctors and have had dozens, or even hundreds, of blood tests and scans and have acquired numerous, often conflicting diagnostic labels. This is confusing for everyone, but most of all for the patient with ME/CFS. At the same time there are conditions, as we saw in the Introduction, that can be almost indistinguishable from ME/CFS, but which can be relatively easily diagnosed and treated, so it is important to investigate to some degree to rule these out.

What sort of diagnostic investigations are used?

Sadly, there is as yet no validated test for ME/CFS. The diagnosis remains one based on the history, clinical findings and the exclusion of other causes of fatigue, such as anaemia, kidney or liver failure, biochemical abnormalities of calcium or glucose, inflammatory conditions including inflammatory muscle disease, an underactive or overactive thyroid and coeliac disease. We follow the recommendations of the 2021 NICE guidelines, which set out clearly the evidence base for including some tests and not others. The tests recommended in these guidelines include:

- **Blood tests:**
  - Full blood count
  - Kidney function
  - Liver function
  - Calcium and phosphate
  - HbA1c (a test for diabetes)
  - Ferritin (a test for iron deficiency)

- ° Measures of inflammation: the ESR (erythrocyte sedimentation rate) or plasma viscosity (in laboratories that do not perform the ESR test) and the CRP (C-reactive protein)
- ° Creatine kinase (a muscle enzyme)
- ° Thyroid function
- ° Coeliac serology

- **Urinalysis:** To rule out any hidden problem with kidney inflammation that does not show in blood tests. A urine sample should be taken, and a dipstick test done to check for protein or blood.

The guidance suggests that clinical judgement should be used to decide whether additional investigations are required, such as measurements of vitamin D, vitamin B_{12} and folate, serological tests for infections or a 9 a.m. cortisol test to identify an underactive adrenal gland.

> ### Red-flag symptoms
> Occasionally we see people with fatigue who have other signs and symptoms that do not fit well with classical ME/CFS, sometimes known as 'red flags'. If these features are present, more extensive investigation is required. For example, patients with neurological symptoms or signs on only one side of the body could have a brain disorder and may need brain imaging, although this pattern is also seen in functional neurological disorder, which is associated with ME/CFS and is not due to

structural brain lesions. While muscle and joint pains are common in ME/CFS, if there are also signs on examination of swollen joints, or of rashes, hair loss and mouth ulcers, then an inflammatory rheumatic disease or connective-tissue disease needs to be ruled out. In older people, symptoms or signs of heart or lung disease, like exertional chest pain or breathlessness, require further investigation.

Overweight males may have obstructive sleep apnoea, a condition where the walls of the throat relax and narrow during sleep, affecting their breathing. Not only does the condition interfere with getting a good night's sleep, but it also increases the risk of high blood pressure, Type 2 diabetes, heart attack and stroke.

Painful lymph glands are common in ME/CFS, but if a physician finds the glands to be significantly swollen beyond the extent that would normally be seen in an upper-respiratory-tract infection, that would need looking into. Significant, unintentional weight loss would also require further investigation.

Investigations that are not routinely required

The 2007 NICE guidelines also highlighted a number of tests that are *not* recommended because they are of poor discriminatory value. These include:

- **Tilt-table testing**: This is a test to evaluate the cause of unexplained fainting or dizziness. A patient lies flat on a motorized table with a footboard and straps to keep them secure; the table is then tilted to a near-vertical position and heart rate and blood pressure are monitored. Although some people with ME/CFS develop dizziness on standing that is consistent with orthostatic hypotension (low blood pressure on standing), tilt-table testing has not been shown to add to the accuracy of diagnosis of ME/CFS and is both time-consuming and costly. It may be indicated as part of the assessment of severity in someone with ME/CFS.

- **Serological tests**: These are blood tests that look for antibodies that are produced in response to infection. Serological testing is not routinely recommended by a physician unless there is a history of Lyme disease (a bacterial infection spread to humans via tick-bites), HIV or viral hepatitis, toxoplasmosis or acute glandular fever. Even with a proven history of Lyme disease, most people will have been fully treated with antibiotics by the time they see a fatigue centre. There is no evidence after multiple clinical trials that extended antibiotic treatment for Lyme disease is any more effective than a standard three-week course,[9] and a quarter of patients receiving such treatment experience significant adverse effects, including antibiotic-induced colitis and diarrhoea, and allergic reactions.

- **Imaging such as X-rays, ultrasound scans, CT or MRI scans**: There is no routine need in suspected ME/CFS for these.

Exercise physiology testing

Lately there has been a lot of interest in exercise physiology testing in ME/CFS, and reports of abnormalities on repeated exercise testing are said by proponents to discriminate between people with ME/CFS and healthy controls, or people with non-specific fatigue.

One example of this is the cardiopulmonary exercise test (CPET). People undergoing a CPET test are required to exercise to the limit of their tolerance while wearing cardiac monitors and a mask that analyses their levels of exhaled carbon dioxide and oxygen. At present this is an interesting research tool in ME/CFS, which is not without risk of provoking significant post-exertional malaise, and it is not yet sufficiently available or standardized to be of use as a diagnostic test.

CPET does, though, have a clearer role in helping anaesthetists and surgeons to assess a patient's fitness for general anaesthetic and major surgery.

What is the prognosis?

Although there is a wide spectrum of severity of ME/CFS, sadly many people with the condition experience a substantial adverse impact on their occupational, educational, social and personal lives. At worst, this can be to a degree similar to that seen in severe rheumatoid arthritis or multiple sclerosis. Estimates suggest that up to 25 per cent of people with ME/CFS are so seriously affected that they are unable to perform basic personal tasks and are confined to bed or spend the majority of the day there. A significant minority become severely, and sometimes permanently, disabled.[10] A substantial number of people will have a fluctuating course, with periods of near-remission and episodes of relapse.

However, most people diagnosed with ME/CFS will show some degree of improvement over time, especially with supportive multidisciplinary care. The prognosis for adolescents and young adults with ME/CFS is particularly favourable, with full recovery occurring in 75 per cent within two to three years.[11] Our experience is that the outlook for university students is nearly as favourable.

Unfortunately the outlook for adults beyond their mid-twenties with ME/CFS is not so good. One recent UK study of more than 8,000 patients with ME/CFS attending NHS services for the condition, who were followed up for up to twenty months, showed improvements in fatigue, pain, anxiety and depression, but little if any improvement in physical function.[12] A further analysis of the same group, followed for up to five years, showed that while one-third rated themselves much better and one-third a little better, the remaining third were either a little worse or much worse.[13] When asked, 'Do you think that you are still suffering from ME/CFS?', 85 per cent replied yes.

Data from the US is similar: the Centers for Disease Control and Prevention published a review of studies and reported at least partial recovery rates in around 40 per cent, with full recovery being rare, at around 5–10 per cent.[14]

Based on this data from a large number of subjects, we would have to conclude that despite the best available management, ME/CFS is a long-term condition that persists for the majority of adults even after receiving specialist treatment – albeit a condition that they may have learned to cope with better.

The clear implication is that current treatment is inadequate, although in our estimation it is a lot better than nothing, and that further research into disease mechanisms, diagnostics and therapeutics is urgently required.

Another implication, which we believe is important, is that there are people who make a full or nearly full recovery from ME/CFS – somewhere between 5 and 30 per cent, according to the large studies reported above.

The importance of hope

We do not fully understand why some people make a very good recovery. However, while not detracting in any way from the poor life experiences of those with severe ME/CFS, we think it is important to focus on and learn from these individuals. This is partly because, in our experience of supporting people with ME/CFS over the years, the most valuable thing we have to offer our patients is hope. We believe it is vital to the well-being of the patients who consult us that there should be a positive but realistic expectation of improvement over time; and that there is at least a chance of very significant improvement – including full or part-time employment, and a normal or near-normal family and social life – with the right support, even if some symptoms persist.

It is for this reason that we have dedicated a whole chapter to hope, entitled 'Life after ME/CFS', near the end of the book, which features the stories of real patients whom we have treated over the years and who have recovered to varying degrees.

2. PVFS and Other Fatigue-Related Syndromes

When you, or someone close to you, are given a diagnosis of ME/CFS, is it natural to want to turn to the internet for some research.

This can feel overwhelming – just typing ME/CFS into Google returns no fewer than fifty-one million search results. Also, you will probably be struck by the wide variety of labels for the illness, and by the number of conditions said to be associated or linked with it.

In our experience, this can be confusing, bewildering even, both for the person with ME/CFS and their loved ones. And while there are many people with ME/CFS who have websites, blogs, Twitter and Instagram accounts relaying the very latest research findings, these are not always reliable and tend to assume a high degree of familiarity with the conditions described.

We know that navigating this snowstorm of information can be difficult for the newly diagnosed. So that's why, below, we will be summarizing some of the key conditions or syndromes which can overlap with ME/CFS and setting out some of the implications of these for management of ME/CFS.

Post-viral fatigue and post-viral fatigue syndrome

It is very common, after many viruses, for people to take a few days or even a few weeks to recover from the acute symptoms of the infection, such as a runny nose, fever, sore throat or cough.

However, an estimated 10–20 per cent of people will experience persistent flu-like symptoms after these acute symptoms have settled, including malaise, fatigue and lethargy. There appears to be no relationship between the severity of the initial viral infection and the later development of these persistent symptoms.

As this is such a common occurrence and usually resolves by itself, many doctors do not give this a label at all, although some may use the terms 'post-viral fatigue' (PVF) or 'post-viral fatigue syndrome' (PVFS). So PVF/ PVFS is a loosely defined term that simply refers to the normal experience of fatigue after a virus.

Using current classification criteria, a definitive diagnosis of ME/CFS, which can be triggered by a virus, cannot be made until several weeks or months after the onset of symptoms. Not all cases of ME/CFS are caused by an infection, and not all infections that may trigger ME/ CFS are viruses – for example, in the previous chapter we covered the bacteria that cause Lyme disease, Q fever and mycoplasma pneumonia.

Although, sadly, some people with PVFS will go on to fulfil the criteria for ME/CFS, most do not. We do not know the optimal way to manage PVFS to reduce the risk of ME/CFS developing, but it is generally considered that an adequate amount of rest is essential to allow recovery.

Although this is not a well-researched area of medicine, many people who go on to develop ME/CFS after a viral infection report regretting that they rushed back to normal activities, or 'pushed through' their symptoms prematurely.

Hypermobility-spectrum disorder

Hypermobility is a condition where someone can move their joints beyond the normal range of movement. The term 'hypermobility-spectrum disorder' encompasses benign joint hypermobility, benign joint hypermobility syndrome and most of what was previously called Ehlers–Danlos Syndrome type III.

Joint hypermobility is most commonly assessed using a test called the Beighton score.[1] For this test, the subject is asked to perform a series of manoeuvres, illustrated opposite.

A point is given if they are able to perform each manoeuvre, with a score of more than five out of nine in adults, or above six out of nine in children, needed to make a diagnosis of hypermobility.

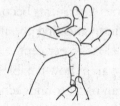

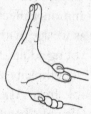

1. Pull little finger back beyond 90 degrees (one point for each side)

2. Pull thumb back to touch forearm (one point for each side)

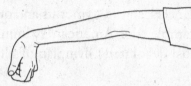

3. Bend elbow backwards beyond 10 degrees (one point for each side)

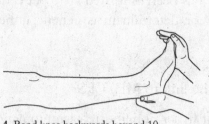

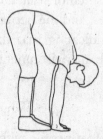

4. Bend knee backwards beyond 10 degrees (one point for each side)

5. Lie hands on the floor while keeping knees straight and bending forward at the waist (one point)

The Beighton score

Are some people more hypermobile than others?

Hypermobile joints are common in childhood and are seen in up to 39 per cent of school-aged children, with girls being more commonly affected than boys. Our joints become less flexible as we age, with the condition affecting about 30 per cent of young adults, falling to below 20 per cent at the age of 60.[2] Our ethnicity also plays a part in how flexible we are, with people from Asian or African backgrounds tending to be more flexible than Caucasians.[3]

For the majority of people with joint hypermobility there is no adverse consequence; indeed, it can be an advantage for dancers, actors, gymnasts and other sports-people. For example, the American swimmer Michael Phelps – the most decorated Olympian of all time – has hypermobility.

There is a strong genetic component to hypermobility, as demonstrated by identical and non-identical twin studies, and the heritability has been estimated at 70 per cent, indicating that the major determinant is genetic rather than environmental.[4]

What is the link to ME/CFS?

Most people with joint hypermobility are asymptomatic, but many of those who have symptoms include fatigue among them, and this can be similar to the fatigue experienced with ME/CFS.

Other symptoms may include experiencing widespread muscle and joint pain, joint sprains and dislocations. Some of these symptoms overlap with ME/CFS and with fibromyalgia.

What's in a name?

Understanding joint hypermobility is made more complicated by frequent changes in naming conventions. Hypermobility without symptoms was until recently referred to as 'benign joint hypermobility', whereas hypermobile people with symptoms were considered to have 'benign joint hypermobility syndrome' (BJHS). Then the syndrome started to be referred to as 'Ehlers–Danlos Syndrome' (EDS) type III, because it appeared to have similarities with other forms of EDS, a group of rare inherited conditions that affect connective tissue. In 1997 a new convention was adopted, and the name changed to EDS-hypermobility type, or EDS-HT.

Meanwhile, genetic studies had been making great headway in finding the causative gene mutations for the many other subtypes of EDS. Some of these subtypes can have very serious adverse health consequences – for example, the vascular form of EDS is associated with sudden arterial rupture and with uterine rupture in pregnancy.

By 2017 thirteen subtypes of EDS had been identified, all but one due to mutations in the collagen gene that controls skin and connective-tissue elasticity. The only one without a collagen mutation identified was EDS-HT. This suggested either that EDS-HT/BJHS is not in fact related to EDS, or that the diagnostic criteria for EDS-HT/BJHS were unduly lax.

Finding the causative gene for any medical condition is akin to looking for a needle in a haystack. One obvious way to make the task more manageable is to shrink the haystack. The best way to do this with a medical condition is to define it extremely tightly, so that only the most definite and severe cases are recruited for genetic studies.

So in 2017, with this in mind, the nomenclature was revised again. Since then the medical label used for those with joint hypermobility not meeting stringent new criteria is Hypermobility Spectrum Disorder or HSD.[5] This label applies to hypermobile individuals with musculoskeletal pain symptoms.

Hypermobile Ehlers–Danlos Syndrome (hEDS)

Also arising from the 2017 revision was a new term for hypermobility thought to represent a subset of EDS. This is now labelled Hypermobile EDS or hEDS. These patients have symptomatic hypermobility and a range of abnormalities, such as leaky heart valves or a widened root of the aorta (the main artery coming from the heart that supplies blood to the trunk, arms and legs). These criteria are deliberately stringent: most hypermobile people with symptoms won't fulfil them.

For the purposes of this book, the most pertinent question is whether hEDS is a cause of fatigue and, if so, whether this meets the criteria for ME/CFS. Another linked question is whether ME/CFS is 'misdiagnosed' in people whose fatigue is actually due to hEDS.

We do not know for certain whether hEDS causes ME/CFS or a related condition, and it is important to note that association and causation are not the same thing. For example, in the 1970s an association between alcohol consumption and lung cancer was found – the more alcohol people drink, the higher their chance of getting lung cancer. Closer examination revealed that, at least at that time, consumption of alcohol and cigarettes went hand-in-hand, and the true cause of lung cancer was not alcohol consumption but the associated cigarette smoking.

Multiple studies have reported fatigue as a common and often disabling feature of hEDS.[6] There is no specific definition for chronic fatigue in hEDS, but it is suggested that criteria similar to those applied to ME/CFS are used, save for post-exertional malaise.

One recent UK study evaluated a small number of patients who had not previously been assessed for hEDS, but had been given a diagnosis of ME/CFS and/or fibromyalgia. They were examined for hypermobility using both the Beighton and the Brighton criteria.[7] The Brighton criteria (unlike the Beighton) consider historical – and not just current – hypermobility. The authors found current or prior hypermobility in 81 per cent of ME/CFS/fibromyalgia patients compared with 37 per cent of healthy controls. This is a significant difference, which suggests association but does not prove causation.

The same symptoms that are often reported in ME/CFS are also reported in hEDS, including:

- Poor sleep

- Chronic pain

- Orthostatic intolerance: feeling faint, or other distressing symptoms on standing

- Headaches

- Anxiety and depression.

Some experts argue that since a diagnosis of ME/CFS requires the exclusion of other conditions causing fatigue, and since hEDS is associated with fatigue, it follows that hypermobile individuals cannot be diagnosed as having ME/CFS, but should be labelled as having hEDS with chronic fatigue.

Yet this seems to us both illogical and hair-splitting, particularly since the management strategies reported as being appropriate for hEDS with chronic fatigue (pacing, multidisciplinary rehabilitation, including occupational therapy, psychology, physiotherapy, pain management, nutritional advice, sleep hygiene) are the same as those commonly used to manage ME/CFS.

Our view, as authors? We believe that ME/CFS and chronic fatigue associated with hEDS are identical.

'Misdiagnosis' of ME/CFS in people with hEDS

The evidence-based treatment for symptoms of fatigue and musculoskeletal pain in the context of hEDS is cognitive behavioural therapy (CBT) alongside physiotherapy.

Experts in hEDS suggest that – unlike ME/CFS, where exercise can trigger PEM – graduated exercise is often helpful for fatigue in hEDs.[8] So it could be argued that if a person is living with ME/CFS in the context of hEDS, they should feel more confident that graduated exercise is an appropriate treatment, based on expert consensus rather than clinical trial evidence.

Non-fatigue symptoms reported in hEDS

Other commonly reported symptoms include:

- **Abnormally stretchy skin**, often associated with stretch marks

- **Heart valve lesions**, such as mitral valve prolapse, but generally not leading to any serious consequence

- **Postural orthostatic tachycardia syndrome (PoTS)**, an abnormal increase in heart rate that occurs after sitting up or standing

- **Orthostatic hypotension**, when the blood pressure drops inappropriately on standing, leading to recurrent faints

- **Irritable bowel syndrome**

- **Structural weakness of connective tissue**, which can lead to rectal prolapse and abdominal hernias in young people.

There are also symptoms that can be associated with the dysfunction of the autonomic nervous system, such as dizziness, fainting, poor concentration, palpitations, brain fog and bladder dysfunction. Some doctors will refer to this as 'dysautonomia'. These symptoms are very common in the general population who do not have hEDS, and expert opinion varies on whether or not it is appropriate to consider them as causally linked with hEDS.

In our opinion, there are significant risks associated with both self-diagnosing and clinician over-diagnosing autonomic failure or dysautonomia.

Finally there is a high prevalence of psychiatric disorder in people with hEDS. In part this may be due to a failure of clinicians to recognize hEDS, and this can lead them to inappropriately ascribe multiple seemingly incomprehensible symptoms to somatization (a tendency to experience psychological distress in the form of physical symptoms). However, multiple studies over the last thirty years have confirmed a striking association between hEDS and anxiety. For example, several studies have found that about 70 per cent of hypermobile people will have anxiety, compared to 10–20 per cent of those who are not hypermobile.[9]

There are also links reported between hEDS and depression, attention deficit hyperactivity disorder (ADHD), autism, personality disorders and eating disorders (some people refer to these conditions as 'neurodiversity', in distinction to the more common 'neurotypical' – this is to recognize that variation from the norm is to be expected and enriches society as a whole). The reasons for these associations are not yet clear, but it is possible that the genes causing hypermobility are also active in the brain, causing structural or other variations that affect brain function and therefore affect the way the mind functions too.

Equally it could be that a heightened sense of interoception (awareness of bodily sensations) – for instance, pain from abnormally lax joint capsules, or a racing pulse due to an increasing heart rate – drive an understandable but counter-productive focus on those sensations, which causes anxiety. Anxiety in turn stimulates the release of adrenaline, which increases the problem of the heart racing and other bodily symptoms.

Fibromyalgia

Fibromyalgia is the term used to describe the combination of widespread pain affecting the spine and all four limbs, with sleep and mood disturbance. An estimated one in twenty adults in the UK has fibromyalgia.[10]

Common symptoms include:

- Pain all over
- Fatigue
- Unrefreshing sleep
- Poor concentration
- Low mood

- Tingling or numbness in the hands and feet

- Headaches

- Restless legs

- Urinary frequency

- Irritable bowel symptoms

- Menstrual pain

- Heightened sensitivity to cold, loud noises and minor trauma.

Many of these symptoms overlap with those of ME/CFS, and indeed studies suggest that 40–80 per cent of people with ME/CFS fulfil the criteria for fibromyalgia, and vice versa.

Diagnosis

Making the diagnosis of fibromyalgia with certainty requires excluding other common causes of widespread pain, such as inflammatory arthritis. Therefore a physical examination and blood tests are required, but the diagnosis is made on the basis of symptoms and an examination to rule out other conditions. There is often, but not always, generalized tenderness in people with fibromyalgia, and finding these 'trigger points' can help in making a positive diagnosis.

Due to this significant overlap with ME/CFS, from a practical point of view, clinicians tend to apply the label fibromyalgia to individuals reporting predominant pain, and ME/CFS to those reporting predominant fatigue. For those who are equally troubled by pain and fatigue, an overlapping diagnosis of ME/CFS/fibromyalgia is appropriate.

Evidence-based treatment in line with 2021 NICE guidelines for chronic primary pain[11] is firstly education, then non-pharmacological approaches such as supervised group exercises, and talking therapies like CBT and Acceptance and Commitment Therapy, named because of its core messages about accepting what is out of your personal control, while committing to actions to improve quality of life.

Another treatment to consider is a single course of acupuncture.

Where pharmacological therapy is necessary, anti-depressants should be offered, such as amitriptyline, citalopram, duloxetine, fluoxetine, paroxetine or sertraline. Where these measures do not provide sufficient relief, a pain-management programme should be considered that includes both physical and psychological components.

It is evident that there is a lot of overlap between ME/CFS and fibromyalgia, many people have both, and their treatment is similar. From a practical standpoint, for us, the main points to bear in mind are that exercise is more problematic as a treatment for ME/CFS because of PEM, and that while there is good evidence that medication can be helpful for fibromyalgia, it is generally unhelpful and more often counter-productive in people with ME/CFS. We generally do not recommend any form of medication to people with ME/CFS unless they are co-morbidly depressed.

Postural Tachycardia Syndrome (PoTS)

Postural tachycardia syndrome, also known as postural orthostatic tachycardia syndrome (PoTS), is a syndrome characterized by frequent symptoms that occur on standing, such as palpitations – tachycardia means 'racing heart' – light-headedness, tremor, generalized weakness, exercise intolerance and fatigue (these are described as symptoms of orthostatic intolerance).

It occurs in around 0.2 per cent of the general population worldwide.[12] It is three times more common in women than in men, and it is more common in people with ME/CFS.

For example, a 2013 UK study of 179 people with ME/CFS found PoTS in 13 per cent of subjects. The affected individuals tended to be younger, with a mean age of twenty-nine compared with forty-two in the non-PoTS group, and they were somewhat less fatigued and depressed than those without PoTS.[13]

It is not clear whether the association between ME/CFS and PoTS is causal or not, or in which direction any such cause operates. It could be that orthostatic intolerance comes first, resulting in the subject becoming unable to tolerate being upright or physically active and therefore developing fatigue secondarily. Alternatively, having to rest as a consequence of ME/CFS might result in the development of orthostatic intolerance.

Either way, PoTS appears not to be the underlying problem in the majority of people with ME/CFS if this study is representative, and it appears to be a decreasingly important aspect as people reach their forties and beyond.

PoTS is also associated with hEDS: a 2020 study looking for hypermobility in a cohort of people with established PoTS found that 31 per cent met the criteria for hEDS, and a further 24 per cent had HSD. This means that, overall, 55 per cent of this PoTS cohort had hypermobility.[14]

The mechanisms underlying PoTS are not clear, but there is some evidence there may be a contribution from autoimmunity, and there seems to be impaired nerve conduction affecting the autonomic nervous system, and a reduced blood volume. There is often poor exercise tolerance ascribed to deconditioning, and this subset of patients has been shown to have reduced heart-wall thickness that improves with exercise training.[15]

There is a higher rate of anxiety in PoTS than in the general population, but the excessive heart-rate response to standing has been shown not to be due to anxiety.[16] Anxiety therefore appears to be a response to, rather than the cause of, the tachycardia, but it is an important aspect of the condition for many, and the treatment of anxiety can be helpful.

Diagnosis

Diagnosis requires the presence of one or more of these symptoms, in addition to an increase in heart rate of more than thirty beats per minute when moving from lying to standing *and* the absence of a significant drop in blood pressure.

Diagnosis also requires measurement of pulse and blood pressure after lying down for a few minutes, then again after standing for a few minutes. There are various protocols suggested, but some take up to twenty minutes, which in most busy clinical environments is simply not practical. A pragmatic approach is to check a recumbent pulse and blood pressure, repeated after standing for three minutes, and if the results are negative for tachycardia but the symptoms are still considered by the clinician to be very suggestive, then a formal tilt-table test (see page 37) should be carried out.

Treatment

Treatment is often difficult; there are no therapies that are reliably effective, and there has been little evaluation by randomized controlled trials. If the symptoms are affecting quality of life, it is recommended that a multidisciplinary approach should be used, including doctors, physiotherapists, occupational therapists and psychologists.[17] Any medication that can worsen PoTS should be stopped.

Blood volume should be increased by drinking 2–3 litres (3½–5 pt) of water per day, and dietary salt intake should be increased to 10–12g per day, if tolerated.

Compression stockings can be helpful. It is recommended that people with PoTS should undergo a regular, structured, graduated and supervised exercise programme featuring resistance training for the thighs. These should initially be restricted to non-upright exercises, such as rowing machines, recumbent bicycles and swimming, until effort tolerance is improved.

Such programmes have been shown to improve symptoms of orthostatic intolerance in military recruits,[18] but have not been formally assessed in people with ME/CFS and PoTS, and in our opinion they are unlikely to be applicable without careful thought and supervision.

There are various pharmaceutical agents that have been suggested to help the symptoms of palpitations, but none is licensed for this indication, and the evidence base for all of them is poor. They include the blood-vessel constricting drug midodrine, beta-blockers like propranolol, selective serotonin reuptake inhibitors like sertraline or citalopram, drugs to increase blood volume such as fludrocortisone, and the stimulant modafinil. All these medications require prescription and supervision by a clinician experienced in managing PoTS, and require regular monitoring of home blood pressure and heart rate.

Mast Cell Activation Syndrome (MCAS)

MCAS is a condition in which people experience repeated episodes of the symptoms of anaphylaxis: a severe, potentially life-threatening allergic reaction. The hallmark of MCAS is recurrent episodes of anaphylaxis with at least two concurrent associated symptoms, including:

- **Cardiovascular symptoms** such as fainting, near-fainting or palpitations

- **Skin symptoms** like urticaria, itching, flushing and angioedema (transient swelling of the eyelids, lips and tongue)

- **Respiratory symptoms** like wheezing and shortness of breath

- **Gut symptoms** such as crampy abdominal pain, diarrhoea, nausea and vomiting.

During these episodes mast cells – the cells that manage allergic reactions within the body – release products called 'mediators'. These mediators include chemicals known as histamine, prostaglandin and leukotriene C4, and must be detected for the diagnosis to be confirmed. Evidence-based guidelines suggest that the diagnosis requires such symptoms to be associated with increases in levels of mast-cell mediators on two or more occasions to establish a diagnosis of MCAS.

Histamine and the other mast-cell mediators are difficult to measure and are not routinely tested. However, specialist allergy clinics can test for serum tryptase and urine markers, including N-methylhistamine. If the diagnosis is confirmed, there is a rationale for using antihistamines to reduce the symptoms.

There have been suggestions that hEDS is linked with

MCAS. While many people state confidently that MCAS, hEDS and ME/CFS are causally linked, this is not established with any scientific rigour – the studies suggesting such a link did not include blood or urine tests to confirm elevated mast-cell products, but were based purely on symptoms.

Moreover, it is not clear that MCAS occurs more commonly in hEDS or ME/CFS than in the general population. Even if it does, it is highly unlikely to occur in more than a small minority of people with hEDS or ME/CFS and so cannot account for the reported symptoms in any but a small minority.

Some have argued that the proposed association with hEDS results from an overlapping pool of vague, subjective symptoms and is inadequate to conclude that any such relationship exists.[19] A 2019 systematic review of MCAS by an expert group of allergy specialists from Harvard University and the Mayo Clinic in the US, and other respected international centres, stated that 'misconceptions about diagnosing MCAS have affected many patients and impaired their quality of life'. It added that disorders that have been used to diagnose MCAS, with no scientific basis for being associated with MCAS, include Ehlers–Danlos syndrome and PoTS, and that use of these disorders to support the diagnosis of MCAS has led to the use of 'unorthodox and potentially harmful therapies'.[20] (You can find out more about allergies in another title in the Penguin Life Expert series, called *Understanding Allergy* by Dr Sophie Farooque.)

While we acknowledge a spectrum of passionately held views, our opinion is that MCAS is over-diagnosed in people with hEDS, PoTS and ME/CFS. In our experience, making the diagnosis does not help the majority of patients that we see, whose main complaint is fatigue, not episodic anaphylaxis.

A thought experiment on physical symptoms and anxiety

To understand the link between anxiety and physical symptoms, let's try something. Think back to the last time you attended a high-stakes examination or interview. Before the event, you will of course have been feeling nervous. As well as having a psychological impact, there will have been physical symptoms. These vary from person to person, but typically include a dry mouth, sweating, trembling, a sensation of butterflies in the stomach and the heart racing or beating hard (palpitations).

We have learned that these are normal physical symptoms to experience when we are nervous, and we know they will settle when the source of stress passes, so we tend only to worry about the stressful event (the examination or interview), and not the physical symptoms themselves.

In long-lasting stress, often we become unaware that we are under strain and instead experience only the physical symptoms of stress, such as palpitations or tremor. These can cause us to worry that something is seriously wrong with our heart or other organs, making us more anxious, which in turn drives more physical symptoms. In these situations, successful treatment of the anxiety can make a huge difference to the physical symptoms and to quality of life.

Healthcare professionals are not immune to these problems. Some years ago, one of us (Gerald) noticed a hard growth between the ribs on his back. It was not painful, but it was enlarging, and he was concerned to have it checked out. He visited a colleague, who after examining him was also concerned and arranged an immediate ultrasound scan of the lump. The radiologist, a good friend of his, appeared very worried, noting that the lump was fixed to the intercostal muscles – the muscles between the ribs. He advised that it could be malignant and that an urgent referral to the regional sarcoma unit should be arranged. Sarcoma is a rare but highly aggressive form of cancer that forms in muscle or bone; it kills a high proportion of sufferers, despite them undergoing what is often life-changing surgery and chemotherapy.

While arranging the referral and waiting two or three weeks for further diagnostic tests and a specialist opinion, Gerald experienced increasing physical symptoms. As well as feeling anxious, unable to concentrate and developing severe insomnia, when he did manage to sleep he would be woken through the night by knife-like pains in the armpits (this is where the lymph nodes that serve the chest wall are located, and they often become enlarged in various forms of cancer). He also experienced nausea, leading to loss of appetite and weight loss. Gerald worried then that he not only had a malignant sarcoma, but that it was already spreading through his body.

When an MRI scan of the lump confirmed that it was in fact a benign tumour – later confirmed, when it was removed – not only was there a massive sense of relief from fear and dread, but the physical symptoms resulting from anxiety disappeared as rapidly as they had arisen, never to return.

3. Theories Regarding Causation

If this chapter were to describe the widely accepted theories of what causes ME/CFS it would be extremely short, because unfortunately, to date, there are none. This is not for any lack of ideas or due to an absence of published scientific research worldwide. Yet for a variety of reasons there have been few high-quality studies of large numbers of people with ME/CFS. Such studies are difficult to design and fund; people who are severely affected and housebound are particularly hard to reach; and the sporadic nature of the condition makes it difficult to find those with early signs of the disease.

In long-term conditions other than ME/CFS, one important aspect of improving scientific understanding has been the study of 'inception cohorts'. This is a rather jargony term, but simply refers to identifying and studying people with early disease. In many long-term conditions, changes occur over time, such as exercise capacity dropping due to pain or fatigue, weight gain for similar reasons, and changes in mood, sleep and hormonal profiles, to name just a few. So simply identifying, for example, 100 people with condition X and comparing them with 100 healthy people is likely to pick up many differences that have nothing to do with disease X's causation, but reflect a correlation with changes that have occurred over time due to living with a long-term illness.

Therefore a recurring theme, when thinking about apparent breakthroughs in our understanding of ME/CFS, is that finding a difference between healthy people and those with ME/CFS is necessary, but not sufficient to demonstrate that such differences are causal (when something is known to definitely cause another thing) rather than merely associated (which could be down to chance).

Another frequent issue is the lack of reproducibility of findings. Over the decades there have been numerous examples of apparent scientific 'breakthroughs' in our understanding of ME/CFS that make it into the world's top scientific journals and into the news headlines, only to be disproved when other laboratories studying different cohorts of people with ME/CFS are unable to reproduce the findings that made the headlines.

One example was the study of a mouse leukaemia-related virus (XMRV), which was reported to be found in the white blood cells of 67 per cent of people with ME/CFS, compared with only 3.7 per cent of healthy control subjects. This study made it into *Science*, one of the world's top journals, and was widely reported at the time.[1] However, after other laboratories could not confirm the findings, and concerns were raised over poor laboratory technique, the paper was withdrawn in 2011.[2]

Similar issues occur when researching many other diseases too, and reflect a variety of factors: lab variation, lab errors or contamination, population variation and sometimes even research fraud. We believe that there are likely to be many papers over the next few years whose authors will claim to have unlocked the secret of ME/CFS and related conditions.

Of course we really hope there *will* be major advances, but we caution that no breakthrough can be considered established until it has been replicated in multiple cohorts, in several countries, and by many independent researchers – this is a high hurdle to pass and, as yet, nobody has succeeded.

Another issue to bear in mind is that most clinicians who have worked with people with ME/CFS believe that it is a heterogeneous disorder. That is to say, while the end result of having ME/CFS is similar, irrespective of the individual's path to the development of symptoms, it is highly unlikely there is a single unifying mechanism causing ME/CFS that holds true for every person with the condition.

For example, some people develop it after a well-characterized infection, but the causative infections are varied – many different viruses and bacteria can be associated with ME/CFS. Others seem to develop it after experiencing persistent inflammatory or autoimmune conditions; and yet others as a result of persistent stress or burnout; and an ME/CFS-like condition is seen in athletes who over-train.

It is difficult to imagine a single cause that applies to each of these cases. As we have already discussed, people with ME/CFS are affected in very different ways – some are able, despite their condition, to work full-time and live a reasonably normal life, while others are housebound or bedbound for years or even decades. This variation in clinical presentation indicates that it is very unlikely that any single causative gene, immunological mechanism or infectious agent is going to explain more than a minority of cases of ME/CFS. That does not mean that we should give up on the search for the causes of it, but it is going to be important to be realistic and not imagine it likely that a scientific 'magic bullet' for the problem is going to materialize in the next five to ten years.

With all these caveats in mind, we still believe it is very important for people learning about their own ME/CFS, or the condition of a loved one, to understand something of the scientific debate about ME/CFS and the landscape surrounding the condition, so that they are in a better position to make sense of any forthcoming potential breakthroughs in the condition.

This reduces the risk that you will be disappointed by false dawns or distracted from the need to confront – with both optimism and realism – the situation you find yourself in. It will allow you to make the best of your situation with appropriate help, without succumbing to a narrative of false hope that might suggest a quick and easy scientific solution is just around the corner.

In the genes? ME / CFS and genetics

There is good reason to think that there is a genetic contribution to ME/CFS. Most long-term illnesses have been found to have both genetic and environmental factors contributing to their development, and it would be surprising if ME/CFS were different. A number of small studies have reported associations between gene variants and ME/CFS, but none have passed the acid test of replication in an unrelated population.

Since 2000 geneticists have been using a different technique, the Genome-Wide Association Study (GWAS), to investigate a variety of conditions (the genome is the entire genetic material of an organism; found in the nucleus of a cell, it is made up of DNA).

This approach requires very large numbers of individuals to be recruited and studied. Unlike earlier 'candidate gene' studies, where scientists choose a gene they think might be involved in a disease and then study variants of that gene in patients and controls, GWAS does not require any prior hypothesis, but rather assesses up to 2.5 million gene variants spread across the entire genome. It is an ideal technique for discovering genetic causes of disease and new biology when the cause is unknown. This is not just because it is comprehensive, but because its results are not influenced by pre-existing hypotheses.

GWAS was important in uncovering, for instance, the novel interleukin 17 inflammatory pathway in a psoriatic arthritis, which led to a new and highly effective medication blocking that pathway.[3]

So it is potentially a significant step that the UK's Medical Research Council has approved and funded the DecodeME study (you'll find a link to this in the Further Reading and Resources section on page 227). This is a

GWAS that aims to recruit 20,000 people with ME/CFS and may reveal genes associated with the condition.

It is clear that if there is a genetic contribution to ME/CFS, it will be polygenic (due to the actions of multiple variant genes) rather than monogenic (a disease caused by variation in a single gene, such as Huntington's disease or cystic fibrosis) – so gene therapy is not going to be applicable.

Moreover, while the study will be important in increasing scientific understanding of ME/CFS, it does not necessarily follow that it will be of very much use in clinical practice. For example, the genes associated with poor outcomes in rheumatoid arthritis have been known since the 1970s, but their discovery has not led to any new therapies; and, as of 2022, genetic testing does not add significantly to the improvement of diagnostic accuracy or the effectiveness of management of rheumatoid arthritis.

Environmental factors

It is likely that, in common with most medical conditions, ME/CFS is the result of environmental factors occurring in a genetically susceptible individual. There are probably several environmental factors that operate, and this section reviews a few of the potential triggers, such as infections, as well as some proposed mechanisms underlying the resulting fatigue.

Infectious agents

There are several viruses that are well known to result in post-viral fatigue in some people, and a proportion of those will go on to fulfil the criteria for ME/CFS. Common examples include:

- **Epstein–Barr virus (EBV)**, which causes infectious mononucleosis (also known as glandular fever)

- **Parvovirus B19**, which causes slapped-cheek syndrome in children and a transient rheumatoid arthritis-like condition in adults

- **Human herpes virus 6, 7 and 8**, which are usually asymptomatic during acute infection.

The mechanisms behind this fatigue are not currently known, but evidence for persistent viral activity as the cause has not been established.

In the 1970s there was a theory that repeated EBV infection caused ME/CFS. This was largely abandoned by the 1990s, due to the ineffectiveness of antivirals and the lack of evidence of viral replication. A pivotal 2022 *Science* paper demonstrated that recent EBV greatly increased the risk of multiple sclerosis, and this will trigger a renewed interest in EBV in ME/CFS.[4]

A number of bacterial infections are also notorious for resulting in significant post-infectious fatigue. These include:

- *Mycoplasma pneumoniae*, which causes pneumonia

- *Borrelia burgdorferi*, which causes Lyme disease

- *Coxiella burnetii*, which causes Q fever, a bacterial infection that you can catch from infected farm animals.

One hypothesis for the continued fatigue after these bacterial infections is that there is some persistent infection driving the fatigue. Since antibiotics are available and effective for bacterial infections, this hypothesis led to studies assessing whether prolonged courses of antibiotics, aimed at clearing persisting infection, would help. Sadly, it turns out that they do not, either in Lyme disease[5] or in Q fever.[6] These negative results also make it unlikely that persisting chronic infection is the cause of fatigue in ME/CFS following these bacterial infections.

Vaccinations

Occasionally we come across people with ME/CFS who believe that their symptoms came on as a result of a vaccination. There is currently no data to support this idea, but equally there is no data proving that it could not be true.

The fact that A (in this case ME/CFS) followed B (vaccination) does not prove that B caused A. However, in our experience, many people find it very difficult to accept that, sadly, bad things can happen to people for no reason, and they look for something to explain why their health deteriorated when it did.

Readers may recall the huge controversy in the 1990s over the measles, mumps and rubella (MMR) vaccine, when a group of parents, supported by the now-discredited physician Andrew Wakefield,[7] believed and argued that their children's autism was caused by the triple vaccination. It is relatively easy to bring together a series of individuals who fell ill after a vaccination and argue that the vaccine was to blame.

Disproving such a link is extremely difficult, though, and requires a huge amount of collaborative international epidemiological research. In the case of the MMR vaccine, it was eventually proved that MMR could not have been the cause of autism in these children, but only after many infants and children had unfortunately been scarred or killed by measles due to an incorrect fear of vaccination.[8]

Our advice is that while all vaccinations have rare complications that can occasionally be serious, the health benefits for those at risk always massively outweigh the potential dangers, otherwise the vaccinations would not get through the regulatory process. While it is of course an individual choice, if asked,

we almost always advise people with ME/CFS to get their routine vaccinations.

Immune-system changes

There are many studies that have reported immune dysregulation in people with ME/CFS. These include increased levels of cytokines (chemical mediators of inflammation) and alterations in the function or numbers of white-cell subsets, known as natural killer (NK) cells and cytotoxic T cells.

Studies on cytokines have been conflicting, and there is as yet no consensus on the role of cytokine abnormalities or white cells in the condition. Sleep disturbance can both initiate and perpetuate changes in immune function, so it is currently uncertain whether any immunological variation in ME/CFS is the cause, consequence or a secondary phenomenon of the condition. A detailed review of the immunological abnormalities reported in ME/CFS lies beyond the scope of this book, but if you are interested in reading more on the subject, we have listed a good overview by Professor Julia Newton in the Further Reading and Resources section on page 227.

Mitochondrial dysfunction

Mitochondria are tiny particles known as organelles, which exist autonomously within almost all living cells – human, animal or plant. They provide energy to cells, which is stored in a small molecule called adenosine triphosphate (ATP). There is a suggestion that ME/CFS may be caused, at least in part, by an acquired mitochondrial dysfunction. And there have been reports of abnormal ATP production, increased mitochondrial damage and impairment of some of the metabolic pathways by which energy is provided.[9]

UK physician Dr Sarah Myhill, and her colleagues, reported and marketed a test called the Mitochondrial Energy Score (MES), which was said both to show mitochondrial dysfunction in all those with ME/CFS and to demonstrate a remarkable correlation between the degree of mitochondrial dysfunction and the severity of ME/CFS.

People found to have mitochondrial dysfunction using this test were then able to purchase supplements from Dr Myhill, which were said to correct the mitochondrial dysfunction. However, a subsequent study by Professor Julia Newton's group demonstrated that the MES was not able to distinguish between healthy people and those with ME/CFS, and therefore should not be offered as a diagnostic test.[10]

Professor Newton has, though, reported evidence of some degree of mitochondrial dysfunction in ME/CFS, although this study was of a relatively small number of patients (thirty-eight) and controls (twelve) and did not include any people immobile due to other medical conditions. So again this requires replication and does not establish causation. In general, while it is tempting to argue – and many do – that mitochondrial dysfunction is the cause of ME/CFS, and of the sensation that many people with the condition describe of feeling like they have a flat battery, from a scientific point of view there is a lot more work to be done before it is clear whether or not mitochondrial dysfunction has any causal link with ME/CFS.

Lactic acidosis

Another area of research into ME/CFS concerns skeletal muscle-cell acidosis, perhaps due to a build-up of lactic acid, which is created during exercise by the metabolism of amino acids in muscle. This idea came from a single influential case report in *The Lancet* in 1984 about a subject with post-viral fatigue[11] who showed early and severe muscle acidification following prolonged exercise. This led the authors to speculate that the basis of the fatigue was abnormal lactic-acid accumulation.

Subsequent studies have varied, but have not consistently replicated *The Lancet* paper's findings, with several finding no abnormality of lactate response. In 1990 a small study of people with ME/CFS after exercise showed significantly elevated blood lactate levels, but a more recent and comprehensive analysis of skeletal muscle in ME/CFS, which measured intracellular pH, lactate concentration and mitochondrial function, showed no evidence of abnormalities in skeletal muscle cells of ME/CFS patients.[12] Again, further work is needed by multiple research groups to clarify the role of lactic acid and other metabolic pathways in ME/CFS.

Hormones and ME/CFS

There has long been interest in the idea that hormonal factors might underlie or explain some or all of the features of ME/CFS. After all, fatigue is a common consequence of endocrine (hormonal) illnesses such as an underactive thyroid or Addison's disease, in which the adrenal gland fails and stops producing cortisol – the body's main stress hormone.

Numerous studies have been published regarding the hypothalamic/pituitary/adrenal (HPA) axis in ME/CFS, but many of these are small and not of the highest quality. While there is conflicting data, there does seem to be a mild reduction in cortisol and an impaired responsiveness of the HPA axis to activation, and a blunting of cortisol responses (we would expect cortisol levels to rise with stressors of various types, such as chronic stress, medication or overactivity of the pituitary or adrenal glands). However, there is no convincing evidence that these changes are specific to ME/CFS, or that they *cause* ME/CFS rather than result from it.

There have been studies of hydrocortisone as a treatment for ME/CFS, and the results were not encouraging. In one study, hydrocortisone or a placebo were prescribed to seventy people with ME/CFS, with modest improvement on a global health scale, but no improvement in fatigue or disability. This came at the cost of significant suppression of the adrenal gland in one-third of the patients receiving hydrocortisone, which is a potentially life-threatening complication.[13]

A second study using a lower dose of hydrocortisone showed a significant reduction in fatigue scores in those given the treatment, and no adrenal suppression.[14] However, the positive effects wore off quickly, and the risks were thought to outweigh the modest benefits from this approach.

Moreover, another UK study of seventy people with ME/CFS who had CBT found improvements in fatigue and disability, as well as an increase in cortisol and restored responsiveness of the adrenal gland to stimulation. The authors of this study suggested that hormone dysfunction in ME/CFS was at least partly reversible by CBT, presumably because this treatment reverses factors such as sleep disruption and high levels of stress, which are probably important in HPA-axis dysfunction.[15]

Currently no hormonal treatment is approved or licensed to treat ME/CFS. We often encounter people with ME/CFS who argue that while their hormonal test results – most commonly levels of triiodothyronine (T3) and thyroxine (T4), which regulate body temperature, metabolism and heart rate – are within the normal range for the general population, they are at the lower end of the normal range. They hypothesize that perhaps before they fell ill their levels were at the higher end of the normal range, and therefore for them their current level is too low and they should receive thyroxine supplements to boost them into the high-normal range.

This argument takes no account of the fact that there is significant variation throughout a twenty-four-hour period, or over days, weeks and months, in many human characteristics, including blood pressure, pulse, temperature and hormones.

Our experience is that this is a blind therapeutic alley, and evidence-based guidelines with lay involvement do not support the use of thyroxine to treat ME/CFS.

Psychological factors

The role of psychological factors in ME/CFS is one of the most controversial areas in all of medicine.

Many people who have lived with the condition, often for numerous years and in its most severe form, object in the most vociferous terms to the suggestion that psychological factors could have anything to do with it.

Many of them have tried psychological therapies and antidepressants and have found they did not help them, so they therefore reject the idea that psychological factors are involved in the condition in general, or at least in their own case. Some believe that because many physicians and psychiatrists consider psychological factors to be important in the condition, ME/CFS has been starved of funding for biomedical research, which would by now – but for this approach – have solved the physical basis of the condition and its cure.

Accepting, as we do, that ME/CFS is a real illness that

affects people apparently at random and can be life-changing, disabling and persistent, we can understand why there are many who dismiss the role of psychological factors. Indeed, considering the large numbers of people throughout the world who have ME/CFS – 250,000 in the UK alone, and an estimated 2.5 million in the US – it is striking that major government- or industry-funded research into the condition has been lacking until very recently. A significant proportion of the published research in the field of ME/CFS has been funded by patient groups, which seems tragic to us, considering that many are unable to work. We accept that it is not beyond the realms of possibility that the popular perception of ME/CFS as a condition with a significant psychological component has contributed to this state of affairs.

At the same time, our experience in clinical practice is that when we see people newly diagnosed with ME/CFS, they are often in a state of distress. This is hardly surprising. Putting ourselves in their shoes, we can imagine how difficult it must be to develop a condition that is potentially highly disabling, persistent and which, for many, reduces or ends their independence and their ability to make a living. To then learn that the condition they have has no diagnostic or confirmatory test, that many people (including doctors) have never heard of it or do not believe in it, and that the guidelines state there is no treatment or cure for it can only be devastating.

Many of the people we see with early ME/CFS have a whole series of entirely rational worries about their situation: have the doctors missed something? Will I ever be well again? Can I still hope for a normal life, including work, having a family, going on holiday? How am I going to explain this to my school/university/employer? Will I be made redundant? How am I going to pay my mortgage? Am I going to end up bedbound for the rest of my life?

Our experience is that concerns like these are common and, indeed, normal. It is also our experience that these rational worries can get out of hand and make the ME/CFS worse, by contributing to a persistent downturn in sleep and mood.

In fact as clinicians who regularly care for people with ME/CFS, we are always on the lookout for the presence of significant mood or sleep disturbance as something that we can treat. We do this not because we believe the fatigue is imaginary, or that psychological therapy will make the fatigue go away, but because anxiety or insomnia triggered by ME/CFS causes a downward spiral in well-being, and very often the development of 'polysymptomatic distress' (a state in which multiple physical symptoms develop simultaneously in someone with high levels of generalized anxiety). Such symptoms are usually, in our experience, highly amenable to psychological therapy, which can bring about major improvements in well-being quite quickly. When we assess new patients with ME/CFS, we try to develop an explanatory model for their situation that makes sense to both patient and clinician. Typically, we consider the 'Three Ps':

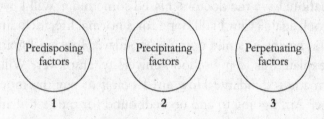

Predisposing factors   Precipitating factors   Perpetuating factors

1   2   3

Theories regarding causation: the 'Three Ps'

Let's return to one of the case studies we considered in Chapter 1 to see how this might work.

You'll recall qualified accountant Nish (see page 28), who had to take time off work after developing work-related stress and anxiety, but had another setback when he caught glandular fever the year after returning to the office. Eventually he had to move back in with his parents and was left bedbound and suicidal.

Let's now use the approach of the Three Ps to look at Nish's case in more detail:

1. **Predisposing factors:** The main predisposing factor in Nish's case would be the episode of depression and anxiety triggered by work stress before he developed a viral illness. We know that a prior history of anxiety and depression does not increase the risk of acquiring a viral infection, but it does prolong the experience of the associated fatigue.[16]

    To be clear, not everyone with a prior history of anxiety or depression suffers post-viral fatigue, and people develop post-viral fatigue and ME/CFS without a prior history of anxiety or depression, but the conditions occur together more often than would be expected by chance.

2. **Precipitating factors**: In Nish's case, the precipitant is clear. He was unlucky enough to acquire an infection with Epstein–Barr virus (EBV) not long after a significant episode of anxiety and depression had made him more vulnerable than he would otherwise have been. EBV is clearly a virus, not a mental-health problem, and had he not acquired this infection, there is no reason to suppose he would have developed ME/CFS.

3. **Perpetuating factors**: It is important to recognize that perpetuating factors are not necessarily the same as precipitating factors, with the result that patients may inappropriately be prescribed antimicrobial therapies that are neither evidence-based nor effective.

One of the most common perpetuating factors that we see (as in Nish's case) is disordered sleep. This is often an accompaniment of ME/CFS, particularly at the more severe end of the spectrum. It can take the form of excessive sleep – we have encountered patients who sleep for more than eighteen hours out of every twenty-four; near-total insomnia;

disrupted sleep, such as sleeping for four to six hours during the day and two or three hours at night; or an appropriate but low-quality, non-restorative sleep architecture.

Not everyone with ME/CFS has these types of sleep problems, but for those who do, CBT can make a big difference, both to their sleep efficiency and ultimately to their fatigue. Sleep efficiency refers to the percentage of time in bed that is spent sleeping, and the most restorative pattern is seen at over 90 per cent. Specifically, for insomnia, CBT is the most effective therapy currently available and is free of drug side-effects and the risk of addiction.[17]

Another feature that Nish's case illustrates is the psychological distress caused by ME/CFS. The overall life expectancy of people with the condition is no different from that of the rest of the population, but sadly there is a sixfold increased risk of suicide.[18] People affected severely by ME/CFS tend, unsurprisingly, to have the highest degree of psychological distress. Seeking and accepting treatment for associated anxiety and depression can help significantly, even though the fatigue persists.

In parallel with Nish's deteriorating mental health, we see a profound deterioration in physical condition, culminating in spending most of his time horizontal. While this is understandable, because the orthostatic intolerance that is a feature of his severe ME/CFS is relieved by lying down, remaining horizontal and avoiding all activity is, unfortunately, only likely to perpetuate his symptoms.

Hypervigilance of physical symptoms does not help, and in fact makes the situation worse – it is for this reason that, in our experience, symptom diaries, sleep apps and wristwatch heart-rate monitors can be a mixed blessing.

While Nish can avoid provoking further deterioration by remaining horizontal, the aim would be that he tries to address his physical inactivity with the support of a multidisciplinary team, as and when he feels ready for it. And while people with ME/CFS are at risk of PEM on activity, there is strong evidence (as we saw in Chapter 2) that orthostatic intolerance – and particularly PoTS – is improved by physical activity, which initially can be done lying down.

Perpetuating factors in chronic musculoskeletal-pain conditions

For both of us, in our clinical practice outside fatigue, we regularly see patients suffering with chronic musculoskeletal pain. Indeed, as we have already discussed, many people with ME/CFS also experience chronic pain as part of their presentation, either because muscle pain is an important feature of ME/CFS, or because they have comorbidities (other simultaneous conditions) such as fibromyalgia or hypermobility spectrum disorder. So what can we learn from these conditions that might apply to people with ME/CFS?

First, distress, depression and anxiety are a common response to any long-term condition, not just ME/CFS, and are seen in around 40 per cent of people with inflammatory rheumatic diseases, such as rheumatoid arthritis, ankylosing spondylitis and psoriatic arthritis. Detecting and treating such mental-health problems is now regarded as best practice in managing these long-term conditions and can make a significant difference to quality of life.

Prognosis for musculoskeletal condition – and, indeed, for many other medical conditions – is influenced quite strongly by psychological factors. For example, musculo-skeletal sprain causing low back pain is a very common condition, affecting 70 per cent of the population at some point in their adult life. This almost ubiquitous phenomenon is precipitated by a physical problem, such as a sprain to muscle, tendon or ligament, but the outcome is determined in large part by the psychological response to the physical injury. Several key beliefs of patients with low back pain have been identified by academics from many countries that predict a poor outcome:

- The belief that back pain is due to progressive disease in the spine.

- The belief that it is harmful or severely disabling.

- The belief that avoidance of activity will help recovery.

- A tendency for low mood and withdrawal from social interaction.

- The expectation that passive treatments rather than active self-management will help.

To identify these beliefs and behaviours is not to diminish or dismiss the pain experience of the person with low back pain: the pain is real. However, the evidence is that if these factors can be identified and addressed, effective rehabilitation will often follow. This is the basis of the advice given these days to people with low back pain – try to keep active and remain optimistic although pain will probably persist to some degree, rather than lie flat for weeks or months until recovery occurs, which was the advice given up until about 1990.

The understanding of these poor prognostic psychological factors also forms the basis of interdisciplinary pain-management programmes, which have doctors, specialist nurses, physiotherapists, occupational therapists and psychologists all working together to help back-pain sufferers improve their function, despite persisting pain. Such programmes have been demonstrated to be more effective than any other form of treatment, including drugs and surgery, in restoring function, even though the original symptom – in this case low back pain – often persists.[19]

A similar approach is evidence-based and is recommended for the management of fibromyalgia and other forms of chronic musculoskeletal pain.[20] The nature and multidisciplinary mix of professionals recommended in programmes to help people with ME/CFS is the same.[21]

Putting our cards on the table, we do not believe that ME/CFS is an imaginary or psychological condition. However, our experience is that while many people cope very well psychologically with their condition and do not need or benefit from psychological treatment, a significant proportion of those who develop persistent or deteriorating fatigue over time show clear evidence of psychological distress and disordered sleep. Supportive treatment by a multidisciplinary team, which addresses psychological factors and guides people through how to manage these, can make a major difference, even though the fatigue usually persists to a greater or lesser degree.

We believe that the systematic identification and treatment of psychological factors in ME/CFS is essential, recommended by evidence-based guidelines (such as the 2021 NICE guidelines), and is not 'medical gaslighting', as some argue. Instead it is responsible, compassionate, patient-centred and, in our experience, very often effective modern clinical care.

4. Self-Management Strategies

'Self-management' is a term used to describe learning and practising a range of skills and strategies to manage our individual health and well-being. This is useful for all of us as we navigate our way through life, but it is particularly helpful for a range of health conditions from chronic pain, to cancer and ME/CFS. Within the context of ME/CFS, learning and using self-management skills can both optimize the chance of recovery and enable an individual to live as full a life as possible with ongoing symptoms.

What is self-management?

During a twenty-five-year career of helping people with ME/CFS, Beverly has always introduced the idea of self-management to people by asking them what they think self-management involves. The answers are varied, and the illustration below sets out the responses she has been given to the question over the years. Take a look at the skills highlighted and consider which of these skills you are already employing in your life. Which do you already find helpful? Which do you feel require some closer attention?

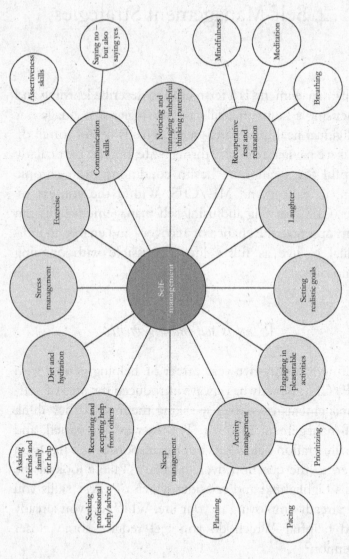

What is self-management?

We'll be discussing many of the terms mentioned in the diagram – such as diet, exercise, sleep and communication skills – a little later on in this book, but for the moment let's focus on the term 'activity management'.

Step 1: Practising activity management

Activity management is a self-management strategy that involves someone with ME/CFS analysing and managing their valued activities: this includes cognitive, emotional, social and physical activity. It is about planning ahead and prioritizing, but it also includes a strategy that many people with ME/CFS cite as being helpful, but difficult to master: pacing. So what does the term 'pacing' actually mean? In its simplest form, pacing describes the different ways of breaking up activities as a means to coping with the impact of your ME/CFS.

To better understand what pacing is, it is worth exploring what pacing *isn't*. The following diagram illustrates what we commonly refer to as peaks and troughs of activity, or boom-and-bust behaviour.

Typically, on a good day when symptoms are less intrusive, it is tempting to do more activity and get things done, perhaps in an attempt to feel 'normal'. At some point during the same day, the day after or even later that week, the symptoms become worse and you are forced to stop and rest. However, this rest period is not really very restful; it is a period of very low or no activity during which you may feel physically and emotionally awful. Symptoms then decline and the temptation to do more returns.

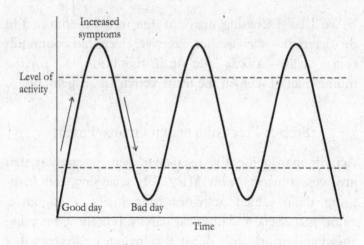

Boom-and-bust behaviour

This boom-and-bust behaviour is driven by symptom severity and leads to significant difficulties in predicting what you will be able to do or what activities you can plan. Pacing, as a general term, means having a more even balance of activities each day, avoiding the peaks and therefore reducing the likelihood of troughs, as shown by the solid line on the diagram. There are various theories and pacing techniques, but in our experience the essential thing is to start by increasing your self-awareness of how you are currently managing your daily activities.

Step 2: Building self-awareness

How do you build self-awareness? We can be terrible historians of our own lives. If we are having a bad day, we may review the whole week in retrospect as being awful and feel as though we did not achieve anything. If we are having a good day, we may remember all of the positive things that we did during the week. Therefore it is important to have some way of recording what we *actually* do, then contemplate why we do these things, before beginning to experiment with doing them differently.

The most common way of doing this is by keeping a diary. Beverly generally asks people to log what they are doing each hour of the day for a week: this must include physical, mental and social activities, rest and, of course, sleep. Using different colours to highlight whether your activities are restful, high-energy or low-energy may help you to see patterns in your day or week. Beverly would suggest using green for rest, red for high-energy and yellow for low-energy; and if you want a medium-energy category, use orange. Categorizing your activities is a very personal thing; for example, I find sitting at the computer filling out a spreadsheet very high-energy, but my twenty-two-year-old son says it is low-energy for him. In addition, watching a TV show that you are not really engaged in may be low-energy, but watching a psychological drama could be high-energy, while meeting your closest friend for coffee could be low-energy, but meeting a work colleague high-energy. Your diary could look something like this, but with the colours added:

Sample diary format

Time	Monday	Tuesday	Wednesday
Midnight–1 a.m.	Sleep	Sleep	Scroll through phone
1–2 a.m.	Sleep	Sleep	Sleep
2–3 a.m.	Sleep	Sleep	Sleep
3–4 a.m.	Awake, pacing around the house	Awake, ruminating on the day	Sleep
4–5 a.m.	Back to sleep	Sleep	Sleep
5–6 a.m.	Sleep	Sleep	Sleep
6–7 a.m.	Sleep	Sleep	Wake up and take medication Try to stay in bed, resting
7–8 a.m.	Shower and dress	Shower and dress	Get up and make coffee
8–9 a.m.	Have breakfast	Breakfast Drive to work	Rest in front of TV
9–10 a.m.	Take dog for a walk	Work	Rest
10–11 a.m.	Light housework	Work	Get dressed
11 a.m.–Midday	Coffee and rest	Work	Empty dishwasher, tidy up
Midday–1 p.m.	Watch TV	Work	Rest

1–2 p.m.	Prepare and eat a sandwich	Lunch break; eat in cafeteria	Eat lunch, then fall asleep
2–3 p.m.	Household admin	Work	Go for a short walk for ten minutes, then rest
3–4 p.m.	Clean the bathroom	Work	Rest
4–5 p.m.	Tea and rest	Work	Read a magazine
5–6 p.m.	Prepare dinner, chopping veg	Drive home Sit with a cup of tea	Watch TV
6–7 p.m.	Partner comes home, chat about the day	Prepare dinner	Prepare and eat dinner
7–8 p.m.	Eat dinner and wash up	Eat dinner and chat	Wash up, rest
8–9 p.m.	Watch TV	Listen to some music	Phone a friend, then rest
9–10 p.m.	Watch TV	Prepare for bed	Watch TV
10–11 p.m.	Prepare for bed	Read in bed	Bed
11 p.m.– Midnight	Sleep	Sleep	Unable to sleep, so scroll through phone

After filling in your activity diary it is useful to ask your-self the following questions:

- Am I taking time to rest during the day?

- What am I doing when I rest?

- How much high-energy activity am I doing before I stop and take a break?

- Do I have some days when I do more than others?

- After a busy day, do I generally have and/or need a quiet day?

- How fixed is my sleep time and rise time?

- Do I sleep during the day?

- Is there any correlation between what I am doing and my need to rest/sleep?

At this point these questions are simply to help you review your daily activities, but the hope is that, with increasing self-awareness, you may then consider making some changes.

Step 3: Committing to making changes

The following case studies of people that Beverly has met aim to illustrate a sense of developing self-awareness and then a commitment to making changes.

Peter, 45

Peter has had symptoms of ME/CFS for nine months. He works full-time as an IT consultant, starting work at 8.30 a.m. and continuing until 3 p.m., when he feels utterly exhausted, is unable to continue and often needs to sleep for an hour afterwards. He schedules all meetings in the morning, as this is when he feels his brain is best able to function. He is frustrated that he is seeing no improvement in his symptoms and is worried that his employer will notice.

When Peter filled out the week-long diary it confirmed that he was cramming in all his activity between 8.30 a.m. and 3 p.m., even at weekends. He rarely stopped for a lunch break, often sat for several hours in Zoom meetings and did very little in the evenings.

I asked Peter if he felt that his behaviour was contributing to the fatigue at 3 p.m., discussing with him that he was doing high-energy mental activity for seven hours without a single break. Peter reflected on this and decided to experiment with taking a mini-break every hour, when he would simply stand up and take a screen break for a few minutes. In addition he would take a ten-minute break mid-morning, as well as a one-hour lunch break. He also agreed to book no more than two Zoom meetings in one day.

His fatigue did not immediately improve, but Peter stuck with it and over the following few weeks he gradually noticed that he was less exhausted at 3 p.m.; in fact he started taking another short break at 3 p.m. and could then return to his desk until 4.30 p.m. Over time, he gradually introduced more activity into his evening and reflected that his work–life balance was improving.

Emily, 32

Emily has had ME/CFS symptoms for eighteen months. Prior to their onset she had a full-time job, went to the gym most mornings and enjoyed socializing. She has not worked since onset, and has noted a gradual deterioration in how much physical, mental and social activity she can do.

Emily's diary illustrated a low level of functioning most days, rising late morning, sleeping mid-afternoon for one or two hours and then sleeping again from 9 p.m. She recorded going out on two occasions during the week: once on Saturday night for dinner with a small group of friends, and once midweek when she was having a good day, for a shopping trip. On both occasions she was out for five hours.

I asked Emily if she thought these high-energy activities were impacting on her symptoms. She said they felt okay at the time, but she was surprised at how bad she felt the next morning. She was able to reflect that this was not unusual, following social outings, but she was keen to continue going as she felt it was important for her mental health.

Emily spent a few weeks analysing her activity more closely and acknowledged that there was a correlation between her activities and her symptoms. She agreed to experiment with moderating these activities, planning to go to quiet venues close to home and stay for a maximum of two hours, and see if this made any difference. She still experiences a variance in her symptoms, but feels more aware now of the decisions she is making and more in control of her symptoms.

Sian, 20

Sian has had symptoms for two years. She is in her second year at university, studying history. Her diary illustrated high levels of activity on Monday to Wednesday, with a significant drop-off by Thursday. Friday, Saturday and Sunday illustrated very low-level activity. Sian also noted that her waking time got later as the week went on.

She said that most of her lectures were at the beginning of the week, which was the main reason for the high levels of activity. She also noted that she socialized more on these days, spending time with university friends because she would probably have to rest at weekends. Sian realized that the accumulation of activity during the early part of the week might be contributing to her symptoms later in the week.

She reviewed her timetable and asked her tutors and friends for support in pacing out her week more effectively. Tutors agreed to send her recordings of some lectures, which she could watch later in the week. Friends agreed to visit her close to home at the weekends, and Sian achieved a better balance.

These three case studies detail how increasing self-awareness and committing to making some changes may help. All three used diaries to reflect on their daily activities and were able to notice unhelpful behaviours, then decided what they were comfortable with doing differently. Peter paced his activities throughout the day by taking regular breaks. Emily moderated her high-energy activities to reduce the probability of over-exertion and symptom exacerbation. Sian recruited her friends and tutors to help her spread her activities throughout the week.

Sleep

The case studies above focus on managing daytime activities, but addressing sleep and potentially making some changes will also be an important part of self-management. The sample diary covers twenty-four hours, which enables you to note when you are sleeping. Many of the individuals I work with believe that getting more, good-quality sleep is the key to reducing their fatigue. Whilst I do not think this is the only answer, addressing sleep issues is an essential part of managing symptoms.

I first learned more about sleep in my early twenties, when sleep came easily for me. I was surprised to find that we do not fall into a deep sleep as soon as our head hits the pillow and we do not stay sound asleep all night. Having some knowledge of sleep science has helped me enormously during the different stages of my life when sleep has been more elusive. I found learning about the stages of sleep particularly useful in reducing my anxiety of regularly waking up at 2 a.m. in my early thirties. It is likely that I had had two full cycles of sleep by then and was waking during a shallow stage of sleep, when it is normal to regain consciousness. I stopped being so anxious, could relax in the knowledge that this short period of wakefulness was not impacting on the quality of my sleep and was able to drift back to sleep more easily.

The following diagram illustrates the different stages of sleep:

- **Stage 1**: This is the dozing-off stage and normally lasts only a few minutes. At this stage the body hasn't completely relaxed and we can easily be woken. If you are not disturbed, you will move into Stage 2.

- **Stage 2**: During this stage the body moves into a more relaxed state, there is a drop in temperature and our breathing, heart rate and brain activity all slow down. This stage lasts between ten and twenty-five minutes.

- **Stage 3**: This is when we move into a deep sleep, our heart rate and breathing decreases and the body relaxes even further. This stage lasts between twenty and forty minutes.

- **Rapid Eye Movement (REM) sleep**: The body reaches a state of temporary paralysis of all muscles, except those that control the eyes and breathing. This is the stage when we can experience vivid dreams. The duration of REM sleep increases as the night progresses.

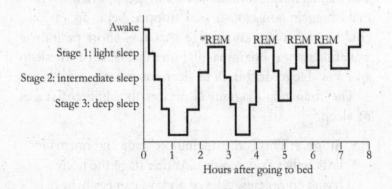

* Rapid Eye Movement (REM) sleep: the sleep phase where dreams occur and the brain is at its most active, processing information and consolidating memories.

A typical eight-hour sleep cycle

The most common sleep-related difficulties that people with ME/CFS experience are:

- Insomnia – difficulty getting off to sleep

- Excessive sleepiness – sleeping for sixteen hours or more out of twenty-four

- Dropping off to sleep during the day

- Sleep delay or even night/day reversal

- Disrupted sleep/frequent waking throughout the night

- A feeling of being unrefreshed on waking.

As with pacing, there is a lot of information available about sleep online. The level of detail that people are looking for varies, but for those who like lots of information we would recommend the Sleep Foundation and sleepOT.org websites (see Further Reading and Resources on page 225), which contain up-to-date information about sleep science, as well as management techniques.

Those who prefer a quick summary of the vast information available about sleep should consider the suggestions below.

Three ways to get a better night's sleep

1. **Set your internal body clock: Going to bed at the same time every night and getting up at the same time every morning will, in time, make it easier to get to sleep and easier to**

wake up. The body learns to expect sleep at a certain time of day, and to be awake at a certain time. Even an hour's shift from your normal bedtime can make sleep more difficult – you may have noticed this when the clocks go back or forward by one hour. It can take up to a week to re-establish our internal body clock. Beverly's husband finds her rigid attitude towards bedtime and wake time very amusing, but her body expects to sleep at 10 p.m. and doesn't like waking up before 7 a.m. Many of the individuals she has worked with also find such rigidity very helpful. Others choose to have a little variation, particularly at weekends. Experiment and see what works best for you. However, make sure you stick with any change in your sleep pattern long enough to work out whether or not it is helpful. Your body clock will also be impacted by light. Try to get some light in the mornings; if you can't get outside, try sitting in a room that gets the morning sun.

2. Optimize your drive to sleep: Increasing your 'drive to sleep' (the likelihood of falling sleep) is controlled by a chemical called adenosine. This builds up during the day when we are awake and reaches a peak approximately fourteen to sixteen hours after waking, triggering the onset of sleep.

Napping during the day will reduce the level of adenosine, so that the onset of sleep at night will be delayed.

3. Wind down before bedtime: The body needs to be in a state of low arousal to have the best chance of sleeping. Worrying thoughts, an argument before bedtime, caffeine, bright light, loud noise, over-stimulation and exercise can all increase arousal, so avoiding these things before bedtime and having a specific wind-down routine will help. And think about the environment you sleep in. Try to make it as comfortable as possible, at the optimal temperature for you. Also try to avoid working in your bedroom – keep it as a place to sleep. It may be important to mention that sex at bedtime can actually help.

Rest and relaxation

The last aspect of self-management that I would like to draw attention to in this chapter is the importance of good-quality rest and relaxation. Incorporating periods of good-quality rest into your daily routine seems like an obvious thing to suggest, but for some people it is very difficult to achieve. As a therapist, when I use the word 'rest' I am referring to resting the body *and* mind, reaching a state of relaxation. However, many of the individuals I work with use this word to describe enforced periods of doing nothing because they are exhausted. Many talk about taking a break from physical activities, but still engage their brains, perhaps by watching TV or reading. I also hear many examples of brains being highly active when they are not diverted by activity – such as thinking, worrying and ruminating – and this state could not be described as rest.

Achieving good-quality rest is a skill that most people need to learn, and it takes practice. There are numerous apps that promise to aid rest and relaxation and we have outlined some worth trying below, including Insight Timer, Headspace, Sleepio and Calm. However, don't expect to feel relaxed the first time you listen. Try out a variety of apps to find the one that suits you – and keep practising.

In addition to trying these more structured ways of resting/relaxing, take a good look at the activities you do and work out which ones are the most restful. Pay attention to how you feel when you do these activities: do you feel relaxed, or perhaps refreshed and energized afterwards? Examples might be watching particular TV programmes, spending quiet time with a good friend, flicking through a glossy magazine, drawing or painting. When you have identified these activities, make sure you prioritize them in your week. Switching between higher-energy activities and these more restful ones can be really helpful.

It is important to recognize that making changes – whether that is managing activity differently, altering sleep patterns or learning how to rest well – is not easy to do alone. Our habits or existing ways of doing things can be hard to change. Friends and family may be able to help, but if you are unable to identify patterns of behaviour or do not notice a positive difference when you make some changes, it may be helpful to seek specialist help. We talk about a referral to specialist services in Chapter 10.

Can apps help me?

As a society, we are increasingly turning to mobile apps and smart trackers to measure everything from what we eat and how we sleep, to our heart rate, mood and stress levels, and the steps we take each day. One analysis found that in 2020 alone, health and fitness apps were downloaded 2.6 billion times worldwide, with consumers spending US $2 billion (£1.5 billion) on paid-for apps.[1]

If you have ME/CFS, then you do need to choose – and use – apps carefully. As we mentioned earlier in the book, hypervigilance of physical symptoms can be unhelpful and may even make the situation worse. Look for apps that can help you with activity management, rather than just symptom tracking.

Here are some apps that we have found to be helpful:

- Headspace uses guided meditations on topics including stress and anxiety management. It teaches techniques around breathing, focus and balance (both free and paid-for content are available via the app).

- Sleepio is an evidence-based, six-week programme that aims to improve sleep with cognitive and behavioural techniques (available on subscription for an online and app programme, but available free of charge to some UK patients on the NHS).
- Insight Timer has more than 80,000 free guided meditations on topics such as stress, sleep and relationships (free and paid-for options are available).
- Calm is another easy-to-use meditation app for all levels, from beginner to advanced, and aims to reduce stress and anxiety (free and paid-for options are available).

5. Treatment Options: Medications and Supplements

It is perhaps unsurprising that people with ME/CFS look to medications or supplements as a way to help symptoms such as fatigue, pain, problems with memory and thinking, as well as countless physical symptoms. You might come across mention of a particular medication or supplement in your own reading, or have the question 'Have you tried . . . ?' posed to you by family and friends, the ME/CFS community or clinicians. The purpose of this chapter is to summarize pharmacological approaches studied in ME/CFS, which we hope will help you assess any such recommendations.

There have been many studies, Cochrane and other systematic reviews examining the effects of graded exercise therapy and cognitive behavioural therapy, and a few on the three-day Lightning Process in ME/CFS, but these are contentious, were reviewed extensively in the 2021 NICE guidelines and are beyond the scope of this chapter.

The placebo response and the role of randomized controlled trials in medicine

Usually the way to demonstrate scientifically that a treatment is effective for a condition or symptom is to carry out a randomized controlled trial (RCT), comparing the potential treatment with a dummy or placebo pill. This is necessary because – regardless of the condition or disease being studied – for most symptoms there is a substantial 'placebo effect' with any intervention.

The placebo effect has been known for decades in relation to medications, and the effect is even stronger for surgical interventions. Let's look at an example. A Finnish study published in the prestigious *New England Journal of Medicine* in 2013 evaluated 146 people with a degenerate and torn knee cartilage, randomizing half of them to have keyhole surgery (at that time one of the most common orthopaedic procedures worldwide).[1] The other half, rather controversially, had sham surgery, in which the subjects were given a general anaesthetic, taken to theatre and had incisions made for the arthroscope (the instrument used to treat the interior of a joint) to be inserted. However, they did not then undergo arthroscopy. Instead the incisions were simply sewn up again, the knee bandaged and the patient woken up.

Neither the assessing clinical team nor the study subjects were told whether they had undergone arthroscopic or sham surgery. To widespread surprise, and not a little disbelief, the Finnish team found not only that the outcome of sham surgery was as good as the outcome of arthroscopic surgery, but also that the benefit was significant in terms of improved pain and function, and was maintained to the end of the study at twelve months postsurgery. From this, we learn that knee arthroscopic surgery for a torn degenerate knee cartilage is no better than sham surgery, but also, surprisingly, that sham surgery gives significant, clinically meaningful and sustained improvement in pain and function.

Now you may wonder why on earth we are discussing the placebo effect of surgery in a book about ME/CFS? Well, partly it is simply to illustrate the powerful effect of any intervention given by a healthcare professional who tries to help someone suffering from symptoms that distress and inconvenience them. This 'placebo response' is both a blessing and a curse. A blessing because it means that any well-intentioned act of professional care is likely to be helpful to people suffering from a health condition, including ME/CFS.

However, the placebo response is also a curse because it makes it extremely difficult to determine whether any improvement in ME/CFS seen after an intervention is a result of the intervention, has happened despite the intervention, or whether the intervention was immaterial in a recovery that would have happened in any event.

This is a problem that applies both to people with ME/CFS who believe that a given intervention helped them to improve – an experience that they then wish to share with other people with ME/CFS – and also to the healthcare professional carrying out the intervention, who typically sincerely believes they are helping.

After all, nobody was more surprised than the orthopaedic community that sham surgery was as good as arthroscopic surgery for people with a cartilage tear in their knee. These surgeons will have received countless heartfelt thanks, boxes of chocolates and bottles of wine from patients grateful for improvements that they experienced after arthroscopic surgery. Such factors are powerful in driving beliefs among patients and clinicians that particular interventions are beneficial, even when subsequent well-designed studies disprove the validity of such beliefs. It also means that clinicians and patients alike would do well to maintain a healthy scepticism regarding anecdotes about interventions that are believed to have helped or hindered people with ME/CFS.

Another reason for mentioning surgery is that some people are reporting fairly drastic surgical interventions as being helpful for their ME/CFS. Several people reported on social media that their ME/CFS was due to a downward herniation of the cerebellum at the base of the brain through the foramen magnum – the hole at the base of the skull through which the spinal cord passes from the brainstem to the spinal canal. In 2019 the American documentary film-maker Jennifer Brea reported that neurosurgery to fuse her cervical spine to the base of the skull completely resolved her ME/CFS.[2]

There was such a flurry of excitement about this that the British ME/CFS charity the ME Association felt compelled to issue an urgent press release[3] pointing out, quite rightly, that such surgery was not supported by the scientific literature, it permanently reduced neck and head movement, was major surgery that carried a significant risk and came at a very high financial cost and, most importantly, had no actual guarantee of helping.

So do any medications 'treat' or 'cure' ME/CFS?

Simply put, there is no high-quality evidence to support any medication as a treatment or cure for ME/CFS. The literature was comprehensively reviewed as part of the 2021 NICE ME/CFS guideline development process, and for those who would like to read an analysis of all the RCTs conducted in ME/CFS, with an overview of their strengths and weaknesses, we recommend reading Appendix F, 'Pharmacological Interventions in ME/CFS' (see Further Reading and Resources on page 224).

While we deplore the state of affairs that sees research into ME/CFS so poorly funded and organized that there is no high-quality evidence to support any intervention, it must also be admitted that this state of affairs is not unique to ME/CFS. There are many medical conditions too rare, sporadic, acute or catastrophic for prospective RCTs to be viable.

For example, several rheumatological conditions have no RCTs to guide their treatment and, in managing these, clinicians do not fall into the trap of therapeutic nihilism – simply stating that there is no evidence for any medication, so therefore we will not attempt any treatment. Rather, as clinicians, we use our best clinical judgement, supported by knowledge from basic science, and from published case studies of patients with the same condition reporting on the results of treatment given in a non-randomized manner.

We also take into account the advice of experts who

see people with such conditions frequently and publish their experiences. This has been drolly characterized as 'eminence-based medicine' – as opposed to the more conventional 'evidence-based medicine' (EBM) that NICE and other bodies espouse. (EBM) is based on systematic reviews and meta-analyses of multiple RCTs. We recognize, therefore, that although there may be individual people with ME/CFS who experience benefit from the judicious use of particular medicines – such as the ones we will cover in this chapter – these medicines have been found wanting in large populations of those with ME/CFS. However, we do not decry such approaches, so long as both patient and clinician are fully informed of the potential risks and the lack of certainty of benefit.

Immunomodulation

An immunomodulator is any drug or substance that has an effect on the immune system. It will either stimulate or suppress the immune system and is used to help the body fight cancer, infection or other diseases. There have been several RCTs of medications that seek to modify the immune response, based on the premise that there may be one or more immunological or autoimmune disorders in ME/CFS. Below we will run through some of these treatments and trials.

- **Rituximab:** This is a targeted cancer drug used in the treatment of leukaemia and lymphoma. It targets and destroys a protein called CD20 on the surface of white blood cells called B-lymphocytes (B-cells). In 2016 a Norwegian group published a series of reports after treating one patient with ME/CFS who developed malignant lymphoma with Rituximab. As well as their lymphoma responding very well to the treatment, the patient's ME/CFS also radically improved. Understandably this generated great excitement, and when later an RCT was organized to compare Rituximab with placebo in ME/CFS, several UK patients were keen to be recruited into it. However, the trial drug was only made available to Norwegian citizens, but in any event the RCT of 151 patients given Rituximab or a placebo showed no additional benefit from Rituximab, although the placebo response was quite impressive, with 35 per cent showing an overall response.[4]

- **Intravenous immunoglobulin (IVIG)**: IVIG is a scarce commodity in healthcare – a treatment derived from the serum of many blood donors, rich in antibodies that can fight infection or reduce inflammation. In the UK it is used in the NHS to treat a variety of immune-mediated or neurological conditions, such as the muscle inflammatory disease polymyositis, the rare post-infectious peripheral nervous system disease Guillain–Barré syndrome, various forms of vasculitis, and paediatric immunodeficiency syndromes. There have been small RCTs of its use in ME/CFS, but none have shown any demonstrable benefit.[5]

- **Rintatolimod**: This drug (also known by the trade name Ampligen) is thought to work by stimulating the body's antiviral pathways and regulating levels of RNase L, a substance found in the cells that helps to attack viruses. Designed with the idea that it could boost cellular defence against viruses and tumours, a 2012 RCT on Rintatolimod found the drug had a modest benefit over placebo.[6] However, regulatory bodies such as NICE in the UK have considered this inadequate evidence of efficacy. It continues to be investigated in the US, but is not approved for use outside a clinical trial.

- **Anakinra**: This is a drug that reduces inflammation by blocking an inflammatory protein called Interleukin-1. A highly effective biological drug, it has transformed our ability to treat a range of serious inflammatory disorders, such as adult-onset Still's disease (a rare type of inflammatory arthritis), familial Mediterranean fever (a genetic disorder that causes recurrent episodes of fever and pain) and the often-fatal inflammatory condition called macrophage activation syndrome, which can affect children with rheumatic disease and is one of the causes of a so-called 'cytokine storm'. A Dutch group investigated the effectiveness of Anakinra versus placebo on fatigue in fifty females with ME/CFS.[7] While 8 per cent of those receiving Anakinra reached a fatigue level within the normal healthy range after four weeks, which seemed promising, the proportion achieving the same while taking placebo injections was better, at 20 per cent. This trial reconfirms the importance of the placebo response and suggests that Anakinra is not useful in ME/CFS.

Antidepressants and antipsychotics

Since mood and sleep disorders often occur in people with ME/CFS, it is not surprising that clinicians have investigated the use of medications that can improve these symptoms. In 2021 NICE reviewed five RCTs for the antidepressants duloxetine, moclobemide and fluoxetine. Three trials compared these agents against a placebo, two others included exercise or graded exercise as well as a placebo. None showed any benefit for sleep quality, activity levels or return to school or work.

Corticosteroids

Commonly known as steroids, corticosteroids are anti-inflammatory medicines used to treat a range of conditions, such as allergies, asthma, eczema and arthritis. In Chapter 3 we briefly looked at some of the evidence for abnormalities in the hypothalamic/pituitary/adrenal axis and some of the trials of corticosteroid for ME/CFS. The 2021 NICE review team identified four RCTs for corticosteroids – one nasal flunisolide, two oral fludrocortisone and one oral hydrocortisone – compared to placebo. In each case they found no evidence of improvement in physical function, activity levels or return to school or work.

Central antihypertensive drugs

Central antihypertensive drugs lower heart rate and reduce blood pressure. They work by blocking signals from the brain to the nervous system that increase the heart rate and narrow the blood vessels. There have been a few reports that the blood-pressure-lowering drug clonidine, which exerts its effect primarily in the brain by stimulating adrenaline receptors, might also help in ME/CFS by lowering activity of the sympathetic nervous system. There are suggestions that it might improve PoTS symptoms and stabilize mast cells. However, in a placebo-controlled RCT it showed no benefit.[8]

Central Nervous System (CNS) stimulants

For many years some clinicians have recommended CNS stimulants for people with ME/CFS. This is based on the hypothesis that daytime sleepiness and problems with cognitive function might be improved by the use of a stimulant, in much the same way that students try to improve their brain power and concentration at exam time using caffeine, modafinil, methylphenidate or other stimulants.

Modafinil has been shown to improve sleepiness that is due to narcolepsy, obstructive sleep apnoea and other sleep disorders, so it seems not unreasonable to investigate its use in ME/CFS. There has only been one small placebo-controlled RCT in fourteen people with ME/CFS, which showed no effect on performance in psychometric tests, or in self-rated fatigue, quality of life or mood.[9]

The CNS stimulants methylphenidate, dexamfetamine and lisdexamfetamine are approved in the UK by NICE for use in attention deficit hyperactivity disorder. A 2005 RCT of sixty patients with ME/CFS treated with meth-ylphenidate showed some improvement in fatigue and concentration in around one in five people with ME/CFS.[10] Then a subsequent study, published in 2018, inves-tigated methylphenidate in combination with a cocktail of vitamins and amino acids verses placebo in 135 people with ME/CFS.[11] While it reported modest improvements in fatigue and concentration, the primary endpoint of change in strength was not significantly dif-ferent from placebo, and NICE considered this to be insufficient evidence of benefit. The data from very small studies of dexamfetamine[12] [13] are not, sadly, much more convincing.

Antiviral drugs

There has long been interest in the idea that ME/CFS, often provoked by a viral infection, might be helped by prolonged courses of antiviral therapy. There have been two RCTs of acyclovir, which is routinely used to very good effect to treat herpes zoster infections (shingles). Sadly, in ME/CFS there is no clinically important benefit in relation to symptom scales or activity levels. There is modest evidence for a trend towards greater improvement of fatigue in those treated with oral valganciclovir versus a placebo, but this did not achieve statistical significance, which means that chance cannot be ruled out for this improvement.[14]

Antihistamines

You may already have a stock of antihistamines stashed in your first-aid kit to relieve symptoms linked to hay fever, hives, conjunctivitis or reactions to insect bites or stings. However, as discussed in Chapter 2, there are those who argue – incorrectly we believe – that ME/CFS and EDS are associated with Mast Cell Activation Syndrome, and that MCAS might account for many of the symptoms of these conditions. If you follow that argument, there could be a rationale for using antihistamines, since activated mast cells release large amounts of histamine. In a study of thirty people with ME/CFS randomized to two months of the antihistamine terfenadine or placebo, there was no evidence of any therapeutic benefit.[15]

Supplements for ME/CFS

Patients will often ask for advice on the benefits of supplements, including vitamin B, multivitamins and magnesium. Below we look at the evidence.

Coenzyme Q10

Coenzyme Q10 plays an important role in the function of the mitochondria, which are often referred to as the powerhouses of our cells, and in the production of ATP, the energy driver of all cells. It is also an antioxidant that is produced naturally in the body. It is used in high doses to treat people who have mutations in their Coenzyme Q10 biosynthetic genes.

An influential study from Belgium, published in 2009, reported abnormally low plasma levels of Coenzyme Q10 in 44 per cent of people with ME/CFS. Those with the lowest levels appeared to have the worst fatigue.[16] There was no attempt in this paper to take the next logical step, which would have been an RCT to determine whether oral supplementation with Coenzyme Q10 would improve fatigue, but others have studied its use as a treatment for post-viral fatigue after polio and have found no benefit.[17] We see little evidence to support its use in ME/CFS, although our experience is that many people take it. It seems generally well tolerated, although it does interact with warfarin, so those taking this medication should avoid it.

Vitamin supplements

There is evidence from one small study of twelve people with ME/CFS that vitamin B deficiency may be a feature of the condition, with deficits found in pyridoxine, riboflavin and thiamine activity.[18] However, this association does not prove causation, and it has not been demonstrated that replacement of B vitamins improves fatigue in ME/CFS.

There was one study of an oral multi-B vitamin for people reporting 'functional fatigue' that would not clearly meet the criteria for ME/CFS, showing an improvement in symptoms compared with a placebo,[19] although other studies have shown no benefit from the combination of vitamin B_{12} and folic acid, or from a multivitamin/mineral mixture.[20]

Hence there is relatively thin evidence, but perhaps some rationale, for taking oral B vitamins, and our anecdotal experience is that many people with ME/CFS do take multivitamins. There is no data to suggest that Myers' cocktail or other fashionable B-vitamin mixtures given intravenously are effective in treating ME/CFS.

Magnesium

Magnesium is a key mineral used by the body to convert food into energy and regulate the nervous system. Many alternative healthcare practitioners advocate magnesium supplementation for ME/CFS. There was a study in 1991, published in *The Lancet*, comparing twenty people with ME/CFS with twenty controls, finding lower red-blood-cell magnesium concentrations in the patients. Subsequently thirty-two ME/CFS patients were randomized to receive intramuscular magnesium-sulphate injections weekly for six weeks or a placebo.

Of those receiving magnesium, 80 per cent reported feeling some benefit, compared with 18 per cent of those receiving the placebo.[21] On the face of it, this looks quite promising, but the study was short, at only six weeks, and injectable magnesium is not user-friendly or easily available. Furthermore, other researchers have found no magnesium deficiency in people with ME/CFS. We would have to conclude that the evidence for the effectiveness of magnesium supplementation for ME/CFS is thin.

Cannabis-related products

In our experience, numerous people with ME/CFS use cannabis-related products to help with pain or sleep problems. Many report finding it helpful, and some see it as transformative. Indeed one of my former patients, Idan Naor, who was housebound with ME/CFS for many years, believes cannabidiol (CBD) played a key part in his recovery. His journey is the subject of the Penguin book *The Little Book of CBD*.

Currently in the UK cannabis products used as a medicine need a product licence, and the Medicines and Healthcare products Regulatory

Agency has not granted a licence for cannabis use by doctors in treating ME/CFS. CBD oil in its pure form is not a controlled drug, as long as the potentially addictive tetrahydrocannabinol (THC) content is below 0.2 per cent, and this is the product commonly used by people with ME/CFS. There have been no RCTS of CBD oil in ME/CFS, so we have no view on whether or not it is appropriate to use it. Given how little evidence there is for any prescribed medicine in ME/CFS, however, we would not criticize those who are tempted to give it a try.

Our position on the pharmacology of ME/CFS

As we have covered in this chapter, the data is not encouraging of the idea that any pharmacological intervention is useful in treating ME/CFS. We are aware of clinicians who do recommend a variety of medications for their patients, despite the lack of high-quality evidence, and we respect their judgement.

We generally do not recommend any medication specifically to treat our patients' ME/CFS, because the evidence of benefit is weak to non-existent, and many of the medications used to treat problems with sleep, pain or mood only make fatigue worse. However, we do occasionally recommend low doses of the antidepressant amitriptyline for those who have severe insomnia, and it must be taken at least two hours before bedtime to achieve any benefit.

A small minority of those we see with ME/CFS have such a high degree of anxiety, distress and agitation at their predicament that we may recommend an antidepressant known as a selective serotonin reuptake inhibitor (SSRI), such as escitalopram, citalopram, fluoxetine, paroxetine, sertraline or the serotonin modulator vortioxetine, which in the main do not worsen fatigue.

Equally we see many people with fibromyalgia in addition to ME/CFS, and for this group – in addition to CBT, which shows strong evidence of benefit in fibromyalgia – we recommend an SNRI (serotonin norepinephrine reuptake inhibitor). Duloxetine is a reasonable option, due to its pain-relieving properties, and is supported by the NICE guidelines on chronic primary pain.[22] We briefly reviewed some of the medications used in PoTS in Chapter 2, and again we are in general in favour of lifestyle modification rather than medication for people with PoTS in the context of ME/CFS.

People with ME/CFS are often very sensitive to medication, and so, as the NICE guidelines state, where we use medication we start at the bottom end of the dose range and increase it only very gradually, and seldom as far as the maximum recommended dose.

6. Nutrition and Food

Food is fuel, as the saying goes. While a balanced, nutritious diet is undoubtedly important for everyone, it is particularly crucial for people with ME/CFS. Our bodies rely on a variety of nutrients for energy, strength, repair and to support recovery. When we can't get what we need from food, the body simply can't work as well as it has the potential to.

There is not one specific superfood or specialist restrictive diet to follow when you have ME/CFS. Instead it is about aiming for variety and balance. Food should be a healthy, enjoyable and positive aspect of your life, not a battle of restrictive diets or guilt around eating the 'wrong' thing.

The aim of this chapter is to show you what a diverse diet looks like, as well as equipping you with practical tips on planning and preparing simple, nutritious food while living with chronic fatigue, to make eating well as simple, sustaining and appetizing as possible.

What does a good diet look like when you have ME/CFS?

ME/CFS can lead to weight changes, such as weight loss caused by poor appetite, irregular eating patterns and a lack of energy to cook; or weight gain due to a lack of physical activity, poor sleep and reliance on processed foods or so-called 'comfort foods'.

Having a good diet means making sure that you get all the nutrients the body needs to function well and at regular intervals, so that you have a steady energy supply. When you are not getting enough energy, you will experience weight loss, which will compromise your immune system and your body's ability to repair and recover. A great starting point is the Eatwell Guide, as shown overleaf.

As this guide demonstrates, balance is the key. Let's take a closer look at the items on your plate and their benefits:

- **Fruit and vegetables**: A brilliant source of nutrients, and they help to keep our gut microbiome balanced (see page 132). They also add colour, texture and variety to our meals, which is particularly important if you have a poor appetite.

- **Fibre**: This is the part of fruits, vegetables, pulses, beans, nuts, seeds and wholegrains that you cannot digest. Fibre is important for your gut health. It encourages the growth of good bacteria in the gut and adds bulk to your food, making your stools softer to pass and preventing constipation; it also helps you feel fuller for longer.

- **Carbohydrates**: Carbohydrates such as potatoes, bread, rice, pasta and other cereals – especially wholegrain ones – provide fibre and energy. Oats and wholegrains release energy slowly and help to keep your energy levels stable.

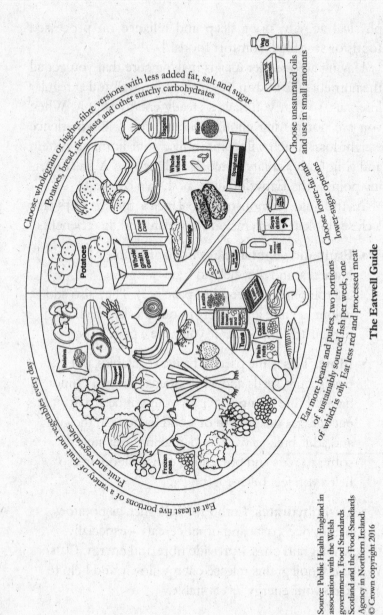

The Eatwell Guide

Choose wholegrain or higher-fibre versions with less added fat, salt and sugar
Potatoes, bread, rice, pasta and other starchy carbohydrates

Choose unsaturated oils and use in small amounts

Choose lower-fat and lower-sugar options

Eat more beans and pulses, two portions of sustainably sourced fish per week, one of which is oily. Eat less red and processed meat

Eat at least five portions of a variety of fruit and vegetables every day

Source: Public Health England in association with the Welsh government, Food Standards Scotland and the Food Standards Agency in Northern Ireland.
© Crown copyright 2016

- **Protein:** This is found in lean meats, fish, seafood, eggs, dairy, pulses, beans, nuts, soya and meat alternatives and is an essential building block throughout the body, from the muscles to tissues. It also helps to make antibodies to fight off infection.

- **Dairy or alternatives:** Our diet is a great source of the mineral calcium, which helps to build and maintain bones (99 per cent of calcium in the body is stored in the bones). Dairy products such as milk, cheese and yoghurt are all rich sources of calcium, and leafy green vegetables, soya beans and nuts also contain some, but in smaller amounts.

- **A small amount of 'good' fats and oils, including omega-3 fats:** These help the body to store energy and absorb vitamins A, D and E.

- **High-sugar, high-fat processed foods:** Cakes, pastry, sweetened drinks, biscuits and savoury snacks should be eaten in small amounts, as a treat only. They often contain little nutrition except for empty calories.

How often should I eat?

This will of course depend on your overall appetite and lifestyle, but we would recommend eating smaller, more frequent meals and healthy snacks rather than large, set meals, to maintain a good reserve of energy.

I (Beverly) often talk to clients about the benefits of 'grazing', particularly if you currently have a poor appetite. This could include quick snacks, such as:

- Dried fruit, nuts and seeds
- Wholegrain crackers with some cheese
- Sliced apple with a peanut-butter dip.

The trick with snacks is not always to see them as treats, but rather as part of your overall sustenance. Of course we all reach for a biscuit or have cake or a muffin with coffee sometimes, but try not to make that choice every single time.

Eating also builds into a wider activity-management programme. A regular eating pattern has a positive impact on the structure of your day, whether it is taking time to prepare food or using a mealtime to stop, have a break and take time to enjoy the food you are eating.

We always advise clients to avoid meals close to bedtime, particularly if poor sleep is an issue. It can take a few hours to digest a full meal, so if your body is busy digesting a huge intake, it can't move on to the winding-down and sleep phase.

Tips for eating well while living with ME/CFS

While a good diet is key, it is not always easy to achieve this when you are living with ME/CFS. The prospect of going to the supermarket, unpacking your shopping, weighing and chopping food and standing over a stove before you can even take a bite is daunting.

However, eating well doesn't mean that you have to cook every meal from scratch – and you shouldn't feel guilty about not doing so. It is really important to factor in fatigue when planning your meals. Here are some tips on planning and preparation, as well as shortcuts you can take to make cooking as efficient as possible.

- **Shop smart:** These days there is far more to supermarket freezer sections than just bags of frozen peas or mixed veg. You can save time by picking up bags of pre-prepared vegetables, such as pre-chopped onions, squashes, peppers and soffrito (a mix of onion, carrot and celery that can be used as a base for soups, stews and Italian dishes). There is also a wide variety of frozen fruits, which can be more economical than buying fresh, especially if you live alone.

- **Don't rule out healthier ready meals:** We often recommend ready-made soups as a quick and nourishing meal, and they can be a good option if you find chewing difficult.

- **Batch-cook:** Pre-preparing a dish or recipe and portioning it out into containers, which can be stored in the fridge or freezer and reheated later, will remove the stress of wondering what to cook for each meal, allowing you to savour the dish.

- **Don't forget tinned foods:** These are good to have on standby for quicker meals. Tinned tomatoes are a fast, healthy addition to lots of dishes, and the humble tin of baked beans makes for a no-fuss, filling meal.

- **Ask for help if you need it**: Often family and friends will ask you what they can do to help, so if you are not feeling up to cooking (or simply don't like doing it), ask them to fill your freezer with pre-made meals.

Look after your gut

The microbiome is the collective name given to the trillions of organisms, such as bacteria, viruses and fungi, that are living and thriving in our gut. Research shows that the microbiome plays a hugely important role in general health, from metabolism and immune function, to disease prevention and good mental health.

Eating a balanced diet encourages the growth of 'good' bacteria, which aids digestion, but also boosts our energy levels. Good bacteria also encourage the production of the chemical known as serotonin in the gut, which can improve mood.[1]

Why hydration is key

It could be argued that hydration is even more important than nutrition. Staying hydrated keeps our kidneys working effectively, whereas not drinking enough fluids can lead to reduced alertness, headaches, brain fog, an increased risk of urinary-tract infections, and even falls in those who are frail.

A good amount to aim to drink is 1.5–2 litres (2½–3½ pt) or 6–8 mugs or glasses a day. Water is best, but if you find the prospect of plain water hard to contemplate, then milk, herbal teas and sugar-free drinks (including tea and coffee) all count. You should limit fruit juice and/or smoothies to a total of 150ml (5 fl oz) a day, due to the high sugar content.

It's also worth bearing in mind that caffeine is a stimulant that can lead to diarrhoea and increase your levels of the stress hormone cortisone. Current advice is to avoid having more than three cups of tea or coffee a day – but it's worth noting that a cup of coffee at home or the office can be much smaller than a large takeaway cup from your local coffee shop.

Remember, though: slowly does it. We all rely on caffeine and sugar at times, so start with small reductions, before building up to larger changes. This advice is about making you aware of the impact that your choices have upon your body so that you are better informed. For example, we've had people arrive in our clinic with a can of energy drink in their hand – this will give you a quick energy fix, but will also send you into an energy slump later in the day.

Vitamins and supplements
A comprehensive multivitamin containing key vitamins and minerals is a good insurance policy, but it is no substitute for a balanced diet. It is better to focus on a Mediterranean-type diet containing lots of fruit and

vegetables, plant-based foods and omega-3-rich food, such as salmon, lean meats and good fats.

As we covered in the previous chapter, there is a lack of evidence on whether magnesium and Coenzyme Q10 supplements help people with ME/CFS. However, one supplement worth taking is vitamin D – this aids calcium absorption and supports strong bones. Known as the 'sunshine vitamin', most of the vitamin D the body needs comes directly from sunlight, mainly during the summer months. UK government guidelines state that everyone over the age of one should get about 10 micrograms (mcg), or 400 International Units, of this vitamin every day.[2] Supplements are important because it is difficult to obtain enough vitamin D from the diet alone, and you may not be getting enough from sunlight if your symptoms restrict how much time you spend outdoors.

Specialist diets and related conditions

Don't underestimate the value of establishing a healthy diet. I remember one client with a dual diagnosis of ME/CFS and irritable bowel syndrome (IBS) who would avoid going out because her trips would be dominated by anxiety about where she could find the nearest bathroom – in case her IBS symptoms flared up. Once she established a food routine that worked for her and helped to ease her symptoms, she regained a sense of control and the anxiety she felt about going out was removed. Before you embark on a special diet, you should always seek professional advice: restricting foods from your diet without sound advice risks depriving your body of vital nutrients and altering your microbiome.

Gluten-free diet

Many with ME/CFS report that their symptoms are helped by following a gluten-free diet. However, there is no research proving this, and current recommendations based on evidence to date (NICE guidelines 2021[3]) do not recommend this diet unless there is a medically diagnosed gluten intolerance, such as coeliac disease. Most gluten-free snacks are more expensive and are actually higher in fats and sugars and calories, and lower in fibre.

Coeliac disease is when people have an adverse reaction to gluten, a protein found in wheat, rye and barley. When they eat gluten, the immune system attacks the tissues in the small intestine, causing damage and inflammation, leaving the body unable to absorb nutrients properly. Coeliac disease affects about one in 100 people in the UK, but in recent years the number of people following a gluten-free diet has grown in prominence: surveys have shown that 23 per cent of people buy gluten-free food, despite not having coeliac disease.

Our advice is that if you suspect you might have an

issue with gluten, see a health professional for tests before cutting gluten from your diet.

Dairy-free diet

Some people with ME/CFS cut out dairy from their diet and report that they are intolerant to milk. Intolerance to milk sugar (lactose) causes gut symptoms such as bloating and diarrhoea. Lactose intolerance is where the body is unable to digest the sugar lactose, found in milk and other dairy products. If you have cut dairy from your diet, then you need to ensure that you are looking to incorporate other sources of calcium in your diet, including: soya or non-dairy alternative drinks and products with added calcium; green leafy vegetables, such as kale and okra; bread or products made with fortified flour. According to UK government guidelines, adults need 700mg of calcium a day. A lack of calcium can lead to osteoporosis, a condition where the bones become weaker and prone to fractures.

Vegan diet

Vegan diets are becoming more popular, with a whole month – 'Veganuary' – dedicated to trying out a plant-based diet. One thing to think about if you have, or are considering, a vegan diet is where you will obtain vitamin B_{12}, which releases energy from food, makes red blood cells and supports the nervous system. A very low B_{12} intake can cause tiredness, anaemia and damage to the nervous system. Adults need 1.5mcg of B_{12} a day, and it can be found in meat, fish, eggs and dairy products. However, it isn't found in foods such as fruits, vegetables and grains, so if you are vegan you need to plan carefully how you will get enough.

Read the labels on food and look for vegan foods that are fortified with B12, including:

- Some plant milks (such as almond, rice or coconut milk)

- Soy products

- Breakfast cereals.

An excellent source of further information and tips to help you achieve a good intake of all nutrients – including B12, calcium, iron – is the Vegan Society website (see page 226).

'Anti-inflammatory' diet

You may have come across this term, although it is simply another name used to describe the well-established and already recommended Mediterranean diet. It is high in fresh fruit and vegetables, lean meat, dairy, good oils, fats and omega-3s, and low in processed foods.

> ### If you have a poor appetite
> If your appetite has waned, or you notice that you are losing weight and find it too much mental and/or physical effort to prepare and eat a meal in one go, you could aim instead for five or six smaller meals a day. It is sometimes easier to boost your nutrition by

having home-made nourishing drinks based on milk or non-dairy milk with flavourings, or smoothies, for example. Another option, available from supermarkets and pharmacies or online, is to buy over-the-counter products that are fortified with vitamins, minerals and protein, such as Complan powder or AYMES nutritional shakes. There are also ready-made drinks such as Fortisip (Nutricia), Ensure (Abbott) and AYMES Complete, which may be more convenient, but these are more expensive.

You can find more information and tips from the British Dietetic Association (see page 225); and the British Association for Parenteral and Enteral Nutrition (BAPEN) has a self-screening malnutrition tool (see page 225).

If you need more help, your doctor can refer you to a dietician for nutritional assessment and support. You will be given help to achieve a good nutritional intake, including other food fortification tips, and you may also be prescribed the varieties and types of nutritional supplements mentioned above, or others.

ME/CFS and IBS

There is an overlap between ME/CFS and IBS. A lot of people with ME/CFS report IBS-like symptoms, such as stomach pain, bloating and constipation and/or diarrhoea. To help with this, try to avoid eating too many gassy foods, such as onions, beans, carbonated drinks and sugar-free gum (which contains an additive that can cause fermentation and produce gas). Avoiding erratic eating and establishing a regular eating pattern will also help. If that fails to settle your IBS-like symptoms, the best next step would be asking your family doctor to refer you to a dietician or accessing one privately.

One option that a dietician may explore with you is what is known as the FODMAP diet, first devised by scientists at Monash University in Melbourne, Australia, and now recommended worldwide to manage IBS symptoms. FODMAP stands for **f**ermentable **o**ligosaccharides, **d**isaccharides, **m**onosaccharides **a**nd **p**olyols. These are short-chain carbohydrates, or sugars, found in a variety of foods, including wheat, some fruits and vegetables, pulses, artificial sweeteners and some processed foods.

Our bodies find FODMAPs difficult to digest. They are poorly absorbed in the small intestine and pass into the large intestine, where they are fermented by bacteria. This produces gas that can cause bloating, wind and pain. FODMAPs can also draw water into the colon, causing diarrhoea. The FODMAP diet is a personalized diet that avoids the specific FODMAPs that can trigger your symptoms, replacing them with alternatives that are easier to digest.

Although this can be very effective, there is much more to the diet than simply cutting out offending foods. It is a complex three-stage process that should only be undertaken with the direction of a dietician to ensure that you are following the diet properly and not missing out on vital nutrients. You can find out more about IBS and the FODMAP diet in another Penguin Life Expert series title, called *Managing IBS* by Dr Lisa Das.

When should I ask for a referral to a dietician?

- If you have a diagnosis of IBS or specific symptoms related to gut health, and efforts to reduce trigger foods haven't worked.

- If you experience weight loss that concerns you: 5–10 per cent weight loss over three to six months is recognized as a risk for malnutrition, so your family doctor should refer you to a specialist for assessment and support.

- If weight gain is affecting your everyday life and recovery.

You can ask for a referral through your family doctor or you can self-refer and see a private dietician. In the UK there is a directory of dieticians organized by specialism, such as IBS or issues with weight loss, to help you find the most suitable professional.

7. ME/CFS, Work and Education

Can work be good for your health? This is a matter of personal opinion. Often friends and colleagues who have no significant health problems will say 'certainly not'. Before we dismiss the idea, however, let's stop for a minute and contemplate what we actually get out of going to work. Financial reward is the obvious starting point, but what else is there? A sense of achievement, a routine, the opportunity to learn new skills and develop knowledge, a feeling of self-worth, making a contribution to society, social interaction, friendship . . . the list goes on.

A 2006 UK government-commissioned report called 'Is work good for your health and well-being?' also found that for people with a health condition or disability, work could have a number of specific benefits,[1] including the fact that work:

- Is therapeutic

- Helps to promote recovery and rehabilitation

- Minimizes the harmful physical, mental and social effects of long-term sickness absence

- Reduces the risk of long-term incapacity

- Promotes full participation in society, independence and human rights

- Reduces poverty

- Improves quality of life and well-being.[2]

Navigating work with ME/CFS

I (Beverly) regularly meet people with ME/CFS who are struggling to sustain work, are on sick leave or have lost their jobs. They recount numerous challenges they have experienced in trying to push through whilst knowing that continuing to fulfil their contracted role is exacerbating their symptoms, and becoming fearful of losing their job due to high absences or lack of perceived capability. These negative experiences obviously impact on self-belief and confidence that working is possible with ME/CFS. However, the challenges that people describe are often related to capacity rather than capability.

For example, capacity barriers can include the ability to work full-time, or sustaining attention for long periods of time, or starting work at 9 a.m. In other words, difficulty doing as much for as long – all of these things can be addressed, though, which we will come to shortly. Let's focus on capability first.

Capability describes what you can do. Think about your work history, skills, experience and talents. These qualities should still be valued, even if your capacity is compromised due to your health. We have worked with teachers, solicitors, nurses, engineers and bankers who all have vast experience and skills to give. Would an employer really want to lose this expertise?

Identifying challenges – and finding solutions

After reminding yourself what you are capable of, the next thing is to realistically identify the challenges that face you. These will be different for each individual, based on your symptoms and your job, but the following table describes some of the most common challenges we have come across with clients, coupled with solutions that have been successfully implemented.

Workplace challenges and their solutions

Challenges (what can increase symptoms)	Solutions (what can minimize the impact on symptoms)
Travelling to work by bus presents challenges, including: • Length of walking time to and from bus stop • Having to stand at bus stop • Possibility of having to stand during rush hour	Negotiate working from home Travel outside the rush hour Apply to the Access to Work scheme (see page 226) for funding for taxis
Distance from car park to place of work beyond walking capacity	Discuss provision of a parking space close to the office

Sustaining attention for prolonged periods leads to increased fatigue	Take regular rest breaks – even a five-minute break will help Use regular screen breaks Let colleagues and managers know you need to stop regularly Split work into forty-five-minute chunks
Workplace lighting is too bright	Request a review of lighting throughout the workplace Negotiate moving to a workspace that avoids bright overhead lights
Workplace is too noisy	Negotiate a quieter space Try noise-cancelling headphones
Full-time work is too exhausting	Request a temporary reduction in hours

Working relationships after an ME/CFS diagnosis

Whether you tell your employer and your colleagues about your diagnosis is largely up to you, but it may be beneficial in the long term to do so. If you are unsure, you should check your contract of employment to see if it specifically states that you must tell your employer about any condition that affects your ability to do your job. Not divulging your diagnosis means that you will be unable to request adjustments that would be helpful – such as asking to work from home because the commute is too tiring.

If you plan to tell your manager about your diagnosis, decide beforehand what you are going to say. Making notes is always helpful. Think about what information your manager needs in order to best support you. This shouldn't be a blow-by-blow account of your medical history, but a succinct factual summary: we would suggest no more than half an A4 page. If you feel the information detailed in any reports from specialists that you have seen is helpful, it may also be worth sharing this.

> **Unsure of what to say – and how to say it?**
> **Chapter 8 contains lots of practical tips on
> how to take ownership of the way you
> communicate your condition to employers,
> colleagues, teachers and classmates so that
> they better understand it, and how you can be
> more assertive so that you get the support
> you need.**

What about telling my co-workers?

As well as your line manager, it also important to consider telling your colleagues. Many people with ME/CFS say they feel guilty about doing things differently and worry that their colleagues will make unhelpful assumptions about why they have been given special considerations.

One primary-school teacher we worked with was exempt

from playground duty, due to her ME/CFS. Breaks were the only time she could find a quiet space to rest, enabling her to return to the classroom and function. She worried that her colleagues would feel put out about having to be on the rota when she was not. Feeling guilty about not taking her turn, she ended up not resting during break time and worrying about people talking about her instead. However, explaining clearly to her colleagues her diagnosis and the reasons why she was exempt from playground duty alleviated this anxiety.

Being upfront with colleagues can change your work experience for the better. For example, if you find sitting in a meeting for two hours without a break both exhausting and painful, let your colleagues know so that you can discuss adjustments – would standing up and moving around at regular intervals help? Could short breaks help to avoid fatigue and pain? You will often find that things that would assist you will help other people too!

Also, think about sharing some ways that you are positively managing your symptoms and how these can be supported at work. For instance, if you find that interspersing your activities with short rest breaks helps your cognitive fatigue and enables you to keep going for longer, don't be afraid to make that known.

Requesting adjustments in the workplace

In our opinion there has never been a better time to request different ways of working. Since the start of the

COVID-19 pandemic in March 2020, employers and employees have had to adapt very quickly to new ways of working, many of which have their advantages.

In the past, many people with ME/CFS and other health conditions have told us that they have requested flexible home-working multiple times, only to be denied, due to lack of IT systems or concerns regarding security. During the pandemic it seems that overnight these concerns disappeared and working from home became the norm.

Of course it may not always be ideal, particularly if you have to share workspace with family members or don't have access to the right equipment, but it does present opportunities to work more flexibly, take regular rest breaks, simply stand and stretch or lie on the floor without attracting attention, avoid rush-hour travel and wear comfortable clothes.

What changes can I ask for?

In the UK employees have a right to request reasonable adjustments to their job; and the employer has a responsibility to consider these adjustments and to ensure that workers with disabilities, or physical and mental-health conditions, are not substantially disadvantaged when doing their jobs.

The 2010 Equality Act defines disability as a mental or physical impairment that has substantial and long-term adverse effects on the ability of a person to carry out normal day-to-day activities.[3] 'Substantial' is more than minor or trivial – for example, if it takes you longer than it usually would to complete a daily task such as getting dressed. 'Long-term' means lasting for twelve months or more.

Under the Equality Act, your employer should make reasonable adjustments to the workplace and to working practices so that you (as a disabled employee or job applicant) are not disadvantaged. Refer back to the chart of workplace challenges and solutions (see pages 143–4) to help you establish what reasonable adjustments you think will benefit you.

What if my employer doesn't agree to the adjustments I request?

In the first instance, it is worth simply having a conversation to try to find out why your employer has said no. In a lot of cases it may be that they simply need more information from you. We would always advise people to seek advice before quoting the Equality Act legislation, as it is important to know whether the requests that you are making are reasonable.

If you are a member of a trade union, contact your local union rep to see if they can help. If you aren't a union member, then the Advisory, Conciliation and Arbitration Service (ACAS, see page 226) is an organization that offers employees and employers free impartial advice on workplace rights, rules and best practice.

If all this feels a little overwhelming (and it's understandable if it does), there are people who can help. Initially we recommend asking your employer or HR department for a referral to an occupational health physician, who will be familiar with a wide range of adjustments and will often know what is reasonable within your specific organization. Specialist ME/CFS services also sometimes have access to therapists with vocational knowledge and experience.

Will a period of time off work help?

If your ME/CFS is overwhelming or workplace stress has been a contributory factor in your condition, then taking sick leave for a period of time may be the only sensible option. However, be aware that the longer the period of time taken off sick, the lower the likelihood of ever returning to work. A period beyond four weeks is described as long-term sickness absence. By the time people have been on sick leave for more than six months, only a minority will ever get back into employment.[4] Given the overwhelming evidence that unemployment has adverse consequences for physical, mental and financial health, we believe strongly that, wherever possible, it is in the best interests of people with ME/CFS to be supported to remain in the workplace, albeit with modifications and a reduction in hours where necessary, rather than going on long-term sick leave.

Returning to work/adapting your working pattern

After you have accessed the support of a multidisciplinary team to optimize your ME/CFS, you may be in a position to increase the duration or intensity of your work to where it was before you fell ill. Clearly, for many people this would be a very good outcome. For some, though, full-time work is possible, but only at the cost of having little or no energy for their life outside work.

We advise people with any health condition that interferes with their work not to make career-altering decisions until they have a definitive diagnosis and have received the best available treatment or rehabilitation, so that they are clear about their likely future capabilities. Having completed treatment with a specialist ME/CFS service, you should be in a better position to make an informed decision about how you balance employment with your health condition and your life outside work.

If a return to work as it was before you developed ME/CFS is no longer viable, other options may include a permanent reduction in hours, altered duties, flexible working, redeployment, seeking a new job or career, or ill-health retirement. Again, your GP, ME/CFS specialist or occupational health physician should be able to help you in making these decisions and in writing the relevant reports that are often required. You could also consider talking to specialist careers consultants to help you with career decision-making.

If you do end up being off work for a prolonged period, do not lose hope. We have known people with ME/CFS who have been off work for more than ten years successfully return to the workplace.

Funding to help you at work

The UK Access to Work scheme was set up in 1994. Essentially this is a pot of central government money to support people with a range of needs to help them get, and stay in, work. The support you receive will depend on your needs, but you can apply and be assessed for:

- A grant to help pay for practical support with your work
- Advice about managing your mental health at work
- Funding to pay for communication support at job interviews.

This practical support might include funding for specialist chairs, desks and computer software, as well as training and mentoring to adapt to your role, transport to and from work, and even physical help from another person with your tasks. Once you have applied you will be assessed to find out what support is most appropriate for you and your work role. Don't worry, you don't need to know what help you want – they are the experts in knowing what is available.

In summary:

- We believe good work is good for you.

- People with ME/CFS can, and do, work. Read the personal stories in Chapter 11 for evidence of this.

- Try to focus on capability, and address capacity by identifying reasonable adjustments.

- Communicate with the people who need to know, and who can help you remain in, or return to, work.

- If needed, access specialist advice and support.

ME/CFS in the classroom

ME/CFS can make children's education challenging for a number of reasons: difficulty concentrating for long periods of time, busy environments and exam stress, to name just a few. However, when it comes to education, many of the same principles as are found in the workplace – communicating with the relevant people, identifying challenges and potential solutions, and negotiating reasonable adjustments – apply.

Why communication is key

We would advise you to communicate with school/college staff as soon as possible. The better your child's teachers understand ME/CFS, the easier it will be for them to make the necessary adjustments. Without information related to the particular symptoms your child is experiencing, and the variability in these symptoms, teachers can make some unhelpful assumptions. I have met many teachers who are confused by the fact that a child can attend one day and present as being well, engaging in lessons and running around the playground, only to hear the next day that the same child is too unwell to attend. You may know this is due to the fact that they over-exerted on the first day, which exacerbated their symptoms, but the teaching staff do not see your child lying on the sofa, feeling exhausted and worrying about missing lessons and their friends.

What adjustments can I ask for?

Some of the adjustments we have discussed with children, young people and their parents include:

- **Having a reduced timetable**: You should bear in mind this may mean reducing the number of subjects studied. I have worked with many teenagers who have reduced their GCSE subjects from ten to six or seven. A reduced timetable will reduce time in lessons, homework, exams and overall pressure. Unsurprisingly, they have found this number of GCSEs to be perfectly adequate!

- **Late or staggered start times**, if early mornings are particularly difficult

- **A quiet place to rest**

- **A 'time out' card** to swiftly alert teachers of the need to take a rest, without having to explain in detail

- **A conveniently positioned locker** to leave heavy books or equipment in

- **A lift key** to enable use of a lift rather than the stairs

- **Access to virtual lessons** and school resources

- **Extensions to homework**

- **Special considerations for exams**.

It is likely that your school will want to formalize any adjustments made to your child's education in a written document. This may include specific details of your child's health and the specialists they are seeing, as well as any adjustments that have been agreed. Websites for the following UK organizations provide up-to-date information on these plans (see page 226–7): the Health Conditions in School Alliance; the Special Educational Needs and Disabilities Information Advice and Support Services; Action for ME.

As with the workplace, the COVID-19 pandemic has revolutionized access to education at a rapid rate. When schools, colleges and universities closed their doors and switched to home-schooling, pupils, teachers and parents alike had to adapt overnight to a new way of working. Virtual classrooms were established, assignments were uploaded rather than handed in, and lessons and lectures were recorded. And for some, this had its benefits: one sixteen-year-old with whom I had worked for more than three years prior to the pandemic was able to access all of her lessons for the first time: no need to travel, no busy corridors, no diverted attention in a noisy classroom. Perhaps hybrid education is a real prospect for the future?

If your child is unable to attend school even for short periods, there are alternative ways of accessing education. Read Hannah's story in Chapter 11 (see page 198) to give you some idea of what this might look like. Hannah's teenage education was not what she or her parents imagined, before she developed ME/CFS. Hannah accessed home tuition, which increased in frequency and duration as she built up her capacity. She was able to take some GCSEs and, after the age of sixteen, attended college. Despite an unconventional route, Hannah is now working in a job she loves.

ME/CFS and higher education

If you or your child had an ME/CFS diagnosis before university, you may well already have strategies in place, and teachers and loved ones will know about your condition. However, university often signals the first move away from the familiarity of the family home, and in new surroundings like university residence halls, lecture theatres and nights out in new places, it can be easy for helpful strategies to fall by the wayside. Again, being upfront and communicating your condition to university staff, course mates and housemates in shared accommodation will be helpful.

It is also worth establishing adjustments early on in your course – ideally, before you even start. Student services in most colleges and universities offer support through a Student Support Plan or Learning Contract, and you should be offered an appointment to discuss your needs if you indicate that you have a disability. The organization Action for ME has some excellent resources on education and ME/CFS (links can be found in the Further Reading and Resources section on page 226). Among the suggested adjustments for students in college and university education are:

- **Longer deadlines** for coursework assignments

- **Additional time in exams**, as well as a separate exam room and breaks

- **Timetabled long gaps** between exams to allow for time to pace revision sessions, and rest days for recovery after long exams

- **Alternatives to timed exams**, such as longer coursework, so that students can demonstrate their knowledge while being able to pace themselves and have breaks.

Funding for university studies

In the UK undergraduate and postgraduate students can apply for a means-tested fund called the Disabled Students' Allowance (DSA, see page 226), to cover the study-related costs due to illness and/or disability. DSA can help with the costs of:

- Specialist equipment, such as computers
- Non-medical helpers, such as a specialist note-taker
- Extra funding to cover travel to attend your course or placement because of your disability
- Other study support: for example, having to print additional copies of documents for proofreading.

8. How Best to Support a Loved One with ME/CFS

'Everyone gets tired – I know I do.'
'You look *terrible* today – I think you need to sit down.'
'Come on, it'll do you good.'

These are just some of the phrases that crop up on a regular basis for people with ME/CFS. Often these comments don't come from perfect strangers, but from those who should know us best, such as partners, children, parents and friends. How you – as someone with ME/CFS – communicate your condition to others is central to the way they will see and support you.

If you have ME/CFS, then the first part of this chapter is for *you*: it will help you think about how to take ownership of the way in which you communicate your condition to others so that they better understand it, and how to be more assertive so that you can get the support you need. The second part, as the title of this chapter suggests, is for those wanting to support a loved one.

It can be difficult to see someone we love struggling to cope. Our natural tendency is to offer help or support, which is commendable. However, you need to be aware of any assumptions you are making in doing this. As well intentioned as your efforts may be, you could end up hindering your loved one rather than helping them. So we also look at practical tips on communication, and establish how best to offer help – as well as what *not* to say – so that you can be the best source of support possible.

Advice for people with ME/CFS

As someone with ME/CFS, you have an important opportunity to develop the understanding that those around you, and closest to you, have about the condition.

Mind your language

The key to developing others' understanding is in how you communicate your condition to them – and that starts with the language you use.

The stresses and strains of everyday life mean that everyone feels tired or fatigued at some point. So when you say to someone, 'I get very tired' or 'I have fatigue' in relation to ME/CFS, the meaning is very often downplayed or misunderstood by those without the condition. When I (Beverly) start working with a client, I will begin by asking, 'How do you put across or communicate what your ME/CFS is?' You don't want to give people a whole essay on your health, but you do want to give them a window into the experience of what it *feels* like to have ME/CFS. To do that, you need to go beyond phrases such as 'I get very tired.'

Some examples of how clients have described their ME/CFS to me in the past include: 'It's a bit like a flu you can't shake off', 'It's like walking through treacle', that their 'limbs feel heavy', or that they 'feel like they have a weighted cloak on their back'. Those with brain fog have described the sensation as a 'muzziness' in their head. I had one client who described ME/CFS as being like having a 'raging hangover and then colliding with a bus'. Extreme, yes, but it absolutely encapsulates how he was feeling at that point.

I work with clients to practise key phrases that they can use when describing their condition to loved ones, colleagues or someone new. We try to use imagery that you can tie into the other person's own experiences, to help form the basis of understanding: 'It's a bit like having a hangover' or 'It's like getting over the flu.' While you might not want to list every single symptom you have, make sure that you communicate the core ones so that the other person is clear on what affects your quality of life the most.

Make sure everyone knows their role, so that they can best support you

Dynamics in families, friendship groups and relationships are built up over decades. Everyone settles into their role as the organizer, the entertainer, the peacemaker or the resourceful one (who is always the go-to person in an emergency). A diagnosis like ME/CFS can turn these established dynamics on their head, so it is important to redraw relationships.

Sit down with your partner, children, parents and friends and be upfront. Have a conversation about how everyone (you included) can improve their communication skills, so that no one is left feeling fed up, offended or misunderstood.

Beforehand you could plan out what you want to say. For example:

- This is my condition.

- These are what my main symptoms feel like and the effect they have.

- This is the reality of the situation, and this is how we can navigate our way through it.

Doing this creates a much clearer method for communicating your condition, rather than simply saying that you feel awful and expecting your family and friends automatically to know how to manage that. Remember, they love you, but you can't expect them to be mind-readers. By all means, you can say that you feel awful, but you should always follow up that statement with 'And this is what I need in order to manage that.'

It's important to explain specifically what you need and how exactly they can support you. A well-meaning parent or partner who is trying to be helpful – but who doesn't actually know what 'helpful' looks like, for you – may end up unintentionally becoming overbearing. Likewise, if you've previously been very independent, then family and friends may think it will irk you to ask if you need help.

This can often be a particular issue in relationships. While some people say their partner intrinsically 'gets' how to act, when to bring them a cup of coffee or offer to take on a task, others will find negotiating this new relationship dynamic very difficult.

The next time someone asks, 'How can I help?', instead of brushing them off, take a moment to think about your answer. Would practical help – such as picking up the children from school, collecting a parcel or doing some gardening – be beneficial for you? Or might a bit of pampering or being taken out for a drive somewhere be what you really need?

Be assertive, not passive

A close friend you haven't seen in a while, who knows you have ME/CFS, invites you for a group evening out. You know, from experience, that the night will likely start with a few drinks down the pub, then dinner, followed by more drinks somewhere else. As you read the message, your immediate feeling is that you are too exhausted. You just can't manage a full-on night out in a crowded pub, loud music, clattering glasses and trying to keep up with multiple conversations. 'They know how tired I get,' you think, 'so why would they even invite me to stand in a busy bar?'

The temptation here is to say nothing about your concerns and simply decline the invitation with no reason offered; or you might decline and offer reams of information on why you can't go. Either response can lead to friction between you and your friends.

You might even accept the invitation without really feeling up to going, worrying that your friends will be offended, or that you will miss out on spending time with loved ones – but you always end up paying for it afterwards. So what can you do? I often ask people to think about their response to invitations like these.

If you want to decline, you could try something like: 'I would really love to go tonight, but you know I have CFS and an evening out is just beyond my current energy levels. You might take a day to get over a hangover, but it could take me two or three days, even if I don't drink any alcohol.'

However, if you do want to go, you can be assertive rather than passively going along with the suggestion or declining altogether. It's about saying to your friends that you do want to come; *however*, you need to make a couple of tweaks to the plans. Instead of declining the invitation outright, you could say: 'I would love to come for dinner with you, but a whole evening out may be too much for me at the moment. Could I meet you all instead for the first hour, before you go on to dinner?'

Or: 'The place you have suggested gets really busy on a Friday night. Could we try somewhere closer to my house, or a place where we can book a table in advance, so I know there will be somewhere to sit when I arrive?'

Or: 'I'd love to catch up with you all, but a big group outing won't work for me right now, so could we try a one-to-one meet-up soon?'

It's about negotiating a way forward that works for you. You should aim to manage the activity yourself, and signal how loved ones can help you. Being honest and looking to adapt the plans means that your friends will not only learn more about your condition, but will also start to offer solutions. You might find that in six months' time the same friend comes to you and says, 'Now I know you might not be up to a full night out, so I've picked this place that is quieter and closer to you, so we can have a good catch-up.'

Advice for supporting someone with ME/CFS

In our experience, supporters tend to fall into two categories. The first is the overly protective – looking out for symptoms, particularly of fatigue, with regular warnings to 'Take it easy', 'You look like you need a rest' or 'Don't worry, I'll do that.'

The second category is the unfailingly positive: 'Come on, it will do you good' and 'Keep on going, you'll be fine', which can make the person with ME/CFS feel irritated and unheard. The support you offer should depend on the needs of the person you are trying to help. You should always start by finding out from them what role they want you to play.

Don't assume you know what's best – ask

It's important that the person you are supporting is given the opportunity to talk about their ME/CFS and how it impacts upon them. You want this to be as relaxed a conversation as possible, so that they feel they can be honest. If you are worried about saying the wrong thing, then ask, 'Is it okay for me to say when I think you need a rest?'

Offer help that is actually *helpful*. 'How can I help?' is a very powerful question, but remember: it involves *actively listening* to the answer.

Many people will appreciate practical help with things like the school run, appointment booking or a bit of housework, but ultimately allow them to decide on the parameters of how best you can support them. If the person says, 'I'm okay' or 'I don't need help', you can try to gently enquire, but if you are met with a flat refusal, then you need to respect that.

Another common approach is for supporters to start meticulously researching ME/CFS. However, before reading reams and reams of research, consult the person you are supporting. Is doing this going to be beneficial for them? If so, is there anything in particular they recommend that you read? Where do they tend to get their information from?

Give them the space to self-manage their condition

It's natural to want to help and it's hard to see someone struggling. Even though friends and family can be fantastic supporters of someone they love who is self-managing their ME/CFS, they can be unwitting saboteurs too.

Let's look at a scenario. Your partner has ME/CFS and is outside doing some gardening. They've been hard at it for most of the morning and you are concerned, so you go out and say, 'Come on, I think you've done enough and could do with a break. Come inside.' Your partner is then irritated because you've told them to stop. They just want to get the job done, so they push themselves even harder to prove that they can. This puts them in an awful mood for the afternoon and you respond with: 'Well, I told you to take a break.'

It's easy to see how exchanges like these can get embedded in your relationship and cause resentment. One way to avoid this is to agree in advance what is going to work and what isn't. Either your partner is on the lookout and decides independently when to take a break, or you have an agreement to go outside and give them a nod when you think it's time for them to have a break – without making a big deal out of it. You don't even have to say anything; it could simply be a gesture like taking them a cup of tea to signal the need to take a pause. Try and avoid beginning conversations with 'I think you . . .' and 'Shouldn't you . . .' Give your loved one the space to self-manage their condition by asserting what they need and what would be helpful.

Another example is at a big social event like a wedding. Rather than wading in with 'I think you look tired and should call it a night', agree the parameters beforehand. It could be that you agree to keep an eye on when your loved one finishes their meal or second drink, so that you can remind them they wanted you to suggest going to a quieter area for a sit-down and a rest. In this case you aren't suggesting a short break because *you* think it is the right course of action, but because you have had permission from your loved one and it is part of them self-managing their condition.

Avoid constant symptom-checking, and try not to make assumptions

How would you react if someone asked you multiple times how you were feeling? Most likely you'd be pretty irritated. Constant symptom-checking, pointing out that someone looks exhausted – or, conversely, full of energy – can be annoying.

Equally, try not to make assumptions about how someone is feeling, based on their appearance alone. They may appear visibly tired or visibly energized, and it's easy to say something like 'You look terrible' or 'You seem full of energy and like you're having a really good day today', but you don't really know how they feel that day.

You will get it wrong sometimes; don't beat yourself up about it

There will be times, despite laying down all the groundwork, when you will say or do the wrong thing – and that's okay. It can be a difficult relationship to manage, so make sure that you take time for yourself, talk to others and find your own support.

9. Questions to Ask Your Healthcare Professional

Living with ME/CFS, particularly in its more severe forms, is a challenge. Given how little is understood about the condition and how to treat it, doctors and other healthcare professionals often find it difficult to know how best to help people with the condition. Mutual misunderstanding and incomprehension are common and can lead to frustration on both sides.

Seeing a doctor about your symptoms is an important step. While it is natural to have a mixture of feelings ahead of your appointment, including some anxiety, remember that seeing a professional is a step towards a clear, definitive diagnosis and having your symptoms recognized and validated. It should also pave the way towards drawing up a plan of management to help you with your symptoms and balancing your work, home and social life.

This chapter is all about helping you to get the best out of a healthcare appointment: preparations you can make beforehand, how to take ownership of the conversation, the things you can expect to discuss and the questions you might wish to ask.

Family doctor or specialist: who should I see?

If you are displaying signs and symptoms of ME/CFS, then your first port of call will probably be a general practitioner or family doctor.

Before the appointment

- **Go ahead and make that appointment:** There is no reason to be embarrassed or feel like you are wasting anyone's time. Healthcare professionals are highly trained, compassionate individuals who are skilled in helping people with all manner of conditions. Any information that you share is confidential.

- **Write it down:** Ahead of your appointment, get into the habit of making a note of the type and severity of your symptoms. Put this information in your diary, on your phone or even record a voice-note, if you prefer.

- **Have a lot to say?** Consider booking a double appointment. The UK has the second-shortest GP appointment times in Europe, according to a 2017 study, with the average appointment lasting just nine minutes. Some surgeries will offer a double-appointment option, but bear in mind that you may have to wait longer to get one. You might also be offered a telephone or virtual appointment (see below for advice).

On the day of your appointment

- **Leave in good time**: When you have to attend an appointment that is important to you, it can make you feel anxious and there is nothing worse than having to rush. Try to reduce stress on the day by leaving plenty of time. Make the appointment your priority of the day – for example, if it is a morning appointment, don't book in anything else beforehand. If you're going by public transport, check the timetable in advance. If driving, give yourself time to get there and find a parking space. In the waiting room take time to ground yourself, so that by the time your name is called you are feeling calm and ready for the appointment.

- **Need some support?** Consider taking a friend. Recalling and absorbing new information during your appointment can take considerable cognitive effort. If you can, bring a friend along to the appointment. If you do this, it is important to discuss and agree beforehand what their role will be. You want them there for support, but the last thing you want is for them to speak *for* you. In our experience, a well-meaning partner or friend will often think they are doing the helpful thing by taking the lead in these conversations, but this can waste valuable discussion time between the patient and the healthcare professional. Think about how your companion can best support you and clearly communicate this to them. Do you need them to prompt you, if you forget something? Should they take notes?

Four ways to make the most of a virtual appointment

The COVID-19 pandemic has had a major impact on how we access healthcare and has prompted a shift towards phone and video consultations. In September 2021 alone, figures show there were 28.5 million appointments in UK general-practice surgeries. While the majority were face-to-face, ten million were telephone appointments, and 140,000 were video consultations.[1]

Don't want an online appointment? Let staff know. Online appointments can be more convenient, but if you don't feel comfortable, then tell a member of staff when booking that you would prefer something face-to-face. Telephone consultations are also increasingly common and have the benefit of being a more familiar form of technology, although this way you lose the visual elements of communication.

Virtual appointments work in exactly the same way as face-to-face ones: a health professional gives advice and you can be referred on to specialist services by them, if needed. But even though many of us will have had plenty of practice on Zoom, Teams, FaceTime and other platforms in our professional and personal lives over the past couple of years, due to the COVID-19 pandemic, if you are given a virtual appointment it pays to do some preparation:

1. Test out the tech in advance: Frozen screens and muted microphones are frustrating all round, so try out a test call with a friend beforehand. Is the room well lit? Can your face clearly be seen? Make use of natural light and try sitting facing a light source (having a window behind you can put your face in shadow). Is the microphone working?

2. On the day of the appointment: Keep a phone close by, in case of connection problems.

3. Clear the room: If you have a partner working from home, ask that they make themselves scarce for the duration of your appointment, as background noise will be distracting for both you and your doctor. If you have young children, try and organize childcare in advance, where possible, so that you can concentrate fully on your appointment.

4. Be on time: Treat a virtual appointment as you would a face-to-face one. Be punctual, do your preparation work and keep any notes or prompts close to your computer.

During your appointment

- **Be succinct**: Even with a double appointment, it is important to be realistic about how much ground you can cover. It isn't the case that doctors don't care, but bear in mind that the typical family GP will see dozens of patients every day, so it is a two-way process to ensure you are getting the most out of your consultation.

- **Short notes are good, printouts not so much**: While it is helpful to make short bullet-point notes, try to avoid coming in armed with reams of paper printed from the internet for your doctor to look over. Sifting through stacks of paper isn't a good way for you or your GP to utilize the limited time in the room together.

- **Take ownership of your health**: You are the expert on how you are feeling. Try to avoid vague statements or long lists. Try and pinpoint exactly what symptoms are affecting your quality of life, and any steps you have taken before your appointment – for example, 'This is what I have done' and 'This is what I need help with.' This will be far more useful than just saying, 'I feel terrible' and 'I don't feel like myself.'

- **Ask questions**: If you aren't sure, ask your doctor to repeat or to clarify. You shouldn't be leaving the room unsure about any advice. For instance, ask, 'What happens now?' or 'How long should I do X for?'

- **Be open-minded**: If the healthcare professional is suggesting something that doesn't fit in with your thinking, try not to dismiss it. Hear them out. While you are the expert in your life and your symptoms, they will have a lot of experience of helping people with diverse medical conditions progress in achieving a diagnosis, getting an appropriate management plan and negotiating a sensible balance between illness and education or work and home life. The relationship between you and your healthcare professional is likely to be most fruitful when both sides respect and trust the other. It saddens us when sometimes we witness or read contemptuous remarks from people with ME/CFS towards their healthcare professionals. While we accept that such attitudes may derive from poor experiences with ill-informed clinicians, our experience is that, ultimately, poor relationships with healthcare professionals are more damaging for the person with ME/CFS than for the clinician.

- **Leave with a plan**: Do you need to book a follow-up appointment? Are you being referred to a specialist? Who should you contact if you have any questions?

10. Referral to Specialist Services

Throughout the book so far we've talked about a number of strategies that we may categorize as self-management or self-help. However, we realize how difficult it is to change habits and beliefs or to implement new good-health behaviours. As human beings, we know that we should eat healthily, drink in moderation and exercise regularly – however, very few of us actually manage consistently to achieve the things we know we need to. Add to this the complications of living with a health condition – particularly one that causes cognitive fatigue – and it's a tall order to live up to good intentions. You will note that in Chapter 11 all of the individuals who agreed to share their stories accessed specialist help.

The aim of this chapter is to look at the type of specialist support available and the therapies that can form the basis of a personalized rehabilitation programme.

What specialist support is available?

The first medical appointment about your symptoms, and the initial step towards a diagnosis, will more than likely be with your family doctor – and Chapter 9 focused on preparation and useful questions that you might need in order to get the best from that appointment.

However, your family doctor may well refer you on to specialist services for more tailored support and a personalized programme. Ideally, those specialist services will consist of an experienced multidisciplinary team. The health professionals you are most likely to find in this team are:

- Occupational therapists
- Physiotherapists
- Clinical and counselling psychologists
- Nurses
- CBT therapists
- Dieticians.

What can I expect at my first appointment?

Your introduction to the service will be with one or two members of the team, whose main aim will be to listen to your story. Please take your time and go prepared with what you would like them to know. This is your chance to educate the professionals not only about your set of symptoms, but also about the impact these symptoms have on your day-to-day life and unique set of circumstances.

It is likely that you will have been sent a set of questionnaires prior to this first meeting. You may feel that you have already covered many of these questions, and the exercise can feel tedious, but it is a very useful way for the therapists to gather information in advance and think about what topics they may want to explore further with you. If you have been keeping activity and sleep diaries, do bring these with you to the meeting as well. They can offer valuable information.

Remember that you will be meeting people who understand chronic fatigue, so if you feel you need a break at any stage, just let them know.

What happens next?

At the end of this appointment, or shortly afterwards, the therapist will discuss options available to you and explain their recommendations. A therapist will base these on scientific evidence, their clinical experience of working with people with ME/CFS and, importantly, your own lived experience. This is your opportunity to ask questions, voice any concerns and make sure that you feel comfortable with what has been recommended.

First steps

Whatever is recommended for you as an individual, the starting point is likely to be a review of your current coping strategies and how effective (or not) these are. Be as honest as you can about how you manage your health – it might be that you are sleeping for long periods in the afternoon, or the only rest you are getting is when you slump in front of the TV at night. Your therapist is not there to make value judgements, but to listen to you and support you in identifying the most effective strategies. They will also explore any difficulties you might be experiencing in making changes or improvements to your health. The idea is that any changes they support you in making will be both achievable and realistic.

What might be in a personalized programme?

Your programme is likely to centre on one or more of the following therapies.

Activity management

You will have the opportunity to analyse your daily routines with a therapist. The therapist may introduce new or unfamiliar strategies, challenge some of your approaches so far and encourage you to experiment with some specific changes. They may give you the confidence to assess, and work on achieving, a balance of cognitive, physical and social activities in your daily life. Some of this may take you out of your comfort zone, but the therapist is there to help you by challenging you and assisting you in understanding and addressing some of the barriers to making changes. These barriers may include guilt, social norms and the internal and external pressure of expectations. Ultimately, this is about finding a manageable balance of activities that are meaningful to you and give you a sense of purpose.

In our experience, once you have found a reasonably balanced range of activities that feel sustainable, it is then possible to increase your level of activity incrementally. This is based on the assumption that periods of rest and recuperation will be incorporated into your daily routine.

Activity management will of course also consider a review of your sleep. If sleep continues to be a significant issue, or your therapist is concerned that you have a sleep disorder, they will help to identify an onward referral to a sleep specialist.

Unfortunately, occasional setbacks (sometimes referred to as flare-ups) are inevitable. Your therapist can help you recognize potential warning signs and manage these times as effectively as possible, moving beyond them, rather than being defeated by them. The illustration below was developed in the pain and fatigue service at North Bristol NHS Trust and is a helpful guide to managing 'the setback pit'.

A note on graded exercise therapy and cognitive behavioural therapy

During the time we have both worked within the clinical field of ME/CFS there has been a lot of debate, with strong opinions on all sides, regarding psychological and physical therapy – more specifically, graded exercise therapy (GET) and cognitive behavioural therapy (CBT). Rather than continue to add to this debate, we would encourage you to go beyond these acronyms and engage with therapists to

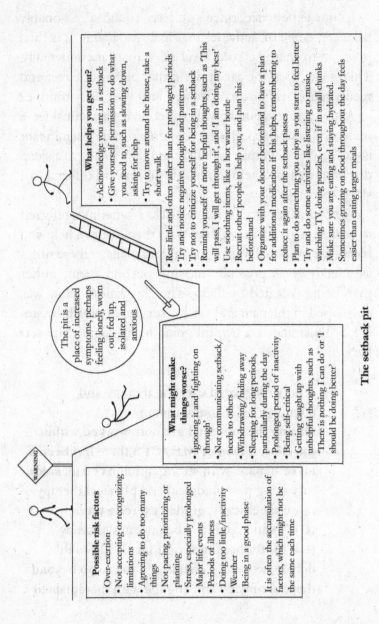

What helps you get out?

- Acknowledge you are in a setback
- Give yourself permission to do what you need to, such as slowing down, asking for help
- Try to move around the house, take a short walk
- Rest little and often rather than for prolonged periods
- Try and notice negative thoughts and patterns
- Try not to criticize yourself for being in a setback
- Remind yourself of more helpful thoughts, such as 'This will pass, I will get through it', and 'I am doing my best'
- Use soothing items, like a hot water bottle
- Recruit other people to help you, and plan this beforehand
- Organize with your doctor beforehand to have a plan for additional medication if this helps, remembering to reduce it again after the setback passes
- Plan to do something you enjoy as you start to feel better
- Try and do some activities like listening to music, watching TV, doing puzzles, even if in small chunks
- Make sure you are eating and staying hydrated.
- Sometimes grazing on food throughout the day feels easier than eating larger meals

The pit is a place of increased symptoms, perhaps feeling lonely, worn out, fed up, isolated and anxious

What might make things worse?

- Ignoring it and 'fighting on through'
- Not communicating setback/ needs to others
- Withdrawing/hiding away
- Sleeping for long periods, particularly during the day
- Prolonged period of inactivity
- Being self-critical
- Getting caught up with unhelpful thoughts, such as 'There is nothing I can do' or 'I should be doing better'

WARNING

Possible risk factors

- Over-exertion
- Not accepting or recognizing limitations
- Agreeing to do too many things
- Not pacing, prioritizing or planning
- Stress, especially prolonged
- Major life events
- Periods of illness
- Doing too little/inactivity
- Weather
- Being in a good phase

It is often the accumulation of factors, which might not be the same each time

The setback pit

explore how psychological therapy (see below) and therapy focused on physical activity (see page 185) might help you.

Psychological therapy

Engaging in psychological therapy does *not* mean that you are imagining your physical symptoms. ME/CFS is a complex illness and, as we have explored, it impacts on many of the body's systems, including the brain. Also, the way you think about the external world and your internal world can have an impact on your mental health and may lead to problems such as anxiety and low mood. This is where a psychological therapy can really help.

Your therapist may base their intervention on different models of therapy. CBT, which we have previously referred to, is summed up in this image:

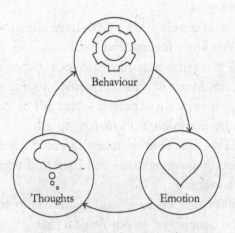

CBT (cognitive behavioural therapy)

However, over the last ten years I (Beverly) have noticed an increase in other psychologically based interventions, such as Acceptance and Commitment Therapy (ACT), Compassion Focused Therapy (CFT) and mindfulness, being introduced into specialist services. These therapies help people develop greater understanding and skills to support them in managing the condition, with a different emphasis to CBT.

Your therapist may not use these specific terms, and may well use elements from a variety of approaches in their work with you. It is worth reiterating that all of us at one time or another would find these therapies of benefit, even without the additional burden of persistent symptoms. Remember that working with any therapist is a collaboration. Together, you can explore what issues are contributing to feelings of anxiety or low mood and, together, you agree on what strategies to employ to make positive changes.

Adults who develop ME/CFS have already had many years of thinking, feeling and behaving. We all develop individual patterns, according to our experiences and environment. Much of this is unconscious and automatic. However, some of these patterns may not be helpful, and may even be detrimental to managing a health condition such as ME/CFS. Your therapist can help you to identify conscious unhelpful patterns and then find ways to make positive changes.

The following two case studies may help to put into context the benefits of psychological therapy.

Julie, 44

Julie had been struggling with significant physical and cognitive fatigue for several years. During our initial sessions she was able to identify that she was caught in a boom-and-bust cycle of activity.

We analysed the reasons that she continued to push herself, even though she knew this would lead to increased symptoms and enforced rest. She was able to recognize that this was largely due to feelings of guilt. She was trying to do things for her family in the way she always had or, in fact, the way she felt a loving mum and wife should do them. She was very critical of herself and felt she was continuously failing to achieve anything well.

Julie agreed to work with one of the clinical psychologists in the team to explore this further. She later told me that this therapy was the key to her changing the way she was managing her activities, and had resulted in a positive change in her symptoms. She said that the feelings of guilt, and thoughts such as 'I should do this' or 'I must just finish this', would still creep into her consciousness, but she could spot these unhelpful thoughts and use the strategies she had learned to avoid falling back into her old automatic responses. She said that she experimented with a range of strategies, but found simply responding to the thoughts with a positive self-statement like 'I am doing the best I can' or 'It is okay to take a break – I can finish this tomorrow' most helpful. These strategies were employed alongside communicating more with her family, redefining her role as mum and wife, learning to rest well and being more compassionate towards herself.

John, 41

John described having significant difficulties in balancing his activities with restorative rest/relaxation. He experimented with scheduling rest breaks into his day, but found that as soon as he sat down and his attention was no longer on an activity, his brain became very busy. He described some recurring thoughts, which included 'I may never feel well again', 'What will I do when my sick pay ends?' and 'Will I lose my job?' These thoughts understandably made him feel anxious, which he recognized prevented him from resting and instead meant that he used up loads of energy.

With the support of his therapist, John worked on defusing these thoughts, distancing himself from them, and instead focused on the present. He practised some mindfulness techniques and gradually found his rest time both recuperative and pleasurable.

Physical therapy

It is difficult to argue with the fact that the body is designed to move. Functional activity, at whatever level, requires strength, stamina, stability and suppleness. For example, even the simple activity of having a shower and washing your hair requires the capacity to step over the side of the bath, stand for five to ten minutes, reach your head to wash your hair, turn off the shower and step out again.

Likewise, a trip to the supermarket requires the capacity to walk, push a trolley, reach up to high shelves and bend down to low ones, lift items out of the trolley onto the conveyor belt and then into shopping bags, which you then need to carry or load into the car. Accessing work may require walking or driving significant distances, climbing stairs and sitting at a desk for prolonged periods of the day.

If these activities are of value to you, and you do not currently have the capacity to do them, it is worth considering getting some specialist advice to incorporate physical activity safely into your daily routine. A skilled therapist who has knowledge of ME/CFS, including PEM, will help you analyse your physical functioning and will work with you to identify activities that will offer benefit, not harm.

If you want to build up your physical tolerance, a physiotherapist or occupational therapist will start by finding out what your baseline level of physical activity is. This is the level that is manageable for you every day, not your personal best. It may include how far you can walk, how long you can sit or stand for or how long you can manage a functional task such as chopping vegetables. As we covered in Chapter 4, our memory of how much we achieve every day may be flawed, and it is better to keep a record of exactly how much you can do.

Many of us now have gadgets that track our movements, or at least our steps. These are helpful for some, but for other people simply timing yourself or counting will suffice. Present this information to your therapist, and you can then discuss how to set your baseline for the activities you are interested in increasing. This may simply be the average that you have managed throughout a normal week, but a baseline can be a bit more nuanced than that and may require a bit more exploration before you get it right. When you have a baseline that you are comfortable with, you can then incorporate it into your daily routine four or five times a week. You are allowed a few days off! If this level is sustainable, you can then discuss a realistic increase with your therapist.

Fiona's story below gives you a sense of how a physical-activity programme can work in practice.

Fiona, 27

Fiona is a young woman who, prior to developing ME/CFS, lived a very busy life. She worked in a financial institution in central London and enjoyed an active social life. Exercise wasn't really her thing, but she did walk twenty minutes to the Tube station each morning and enjoyed dancing.

When I (Beverly) first met Fiona, she was spending most of her day resting on the sofa in a reclined position. On a good day she would occasionally be tempted to go out to a bar or restaurant, which involved walking, sitting and standing for much longer than she was used to, and inevitably she crashed. Fiona chose physical activities to work on: sitting upright and walking. It took us some time to establish baselines, as Fiona started off by completely overestimating what she could do, and her capacity and symptoms continued to fluctuate.

After a number of therapy sessions and lots of record-keeping, Fiona set her initial baselines as ten minutes sitting in an upright chair, and walking around her garden, which took five minutes. Over a period of six months she gradually increased these baselines. There were a few setbacks meaning that Fiona needed to take a step back, which she found very frustrating, but she gradually moved forward. When her walking tolerance reached fifteen minutes she became bored of doing this five times a week, but worked out that if she met a friend who walked her dog daily, this would be a more enjoyable activity.

By the time Fiona completed her rehabilitation programme she could walk for thirty minutes every day and sit for more than an hour, which was sufficient to do the functional activities that were important to her.

<u>Seven ways to get the best out of specialist support and rehabilitation</u>

1. Seek help early.
2. Prepare well for the initial meeting.
3. Be open to what's on offer.
4. Be a partner in the process.
5. Voice any concerns you have at any time.
6. If anything doesn't feel right – including your relationship with the therapist – flag it up.
7. Don't forget that we all need help sometimes.

11. Life after ME/CFS

For many, ME/CFS is a condition that will affect them for life. However, there are people who do make a very significant degree of recovery and return to a life similar to the one they had before they developed ME/CFS. We believe that there is an awful lot to learn from these individuals and their many different pathways to recovery. Throughout both of our careers, working closely with people who have the condition, we have seen at first hand the power that hope has for patients. Encouraging them to retain a belief that things can, and will, improve and that they will enjoy a good quality of life again is crucial. ME/CFS can be an incredibly isolating and daunting condition, and it is often the case that negative stories are much easier to find online, or hear about, than positive ones.

So, very early on during the writing of this book, we resolved to end it with some empowering stories of hope. Below, people who have been through ME/CFS share – in their own words – their stories of recovery, in the hope that their experiences will bring a fresh sense of optimism to others.

James, 42

'I first developed symptoms in 2017. I'd had a serious heart infection about nine months before, and the next time I got ill I seemed unable to recover – I was becoming increasingly tired and having to rest more and more. This gradually evolved into a whole series of physical symptoms, from exhaustion, breathlessness, feeling dizzy and dissociation, to an inability to stand for very long, anxiety and palpitations.

'As a lawyer and father of two young children, I was used to always being busy, and I loved exercise. But I was floored by my symptoms. I was referred to a specialist fatigue clinic via my family doctor and was then diagnosed with ME/CFS. The diagnosis was a revelation, as by that point I wasn't sure anyone would be able to tell me what was wrong. It was explained to me that effectively my fight-or-flight reaction had got stuck and was always turned on.

'For me, CBT and meditation have been vital. I started off using the Headspace meditation app, and I took up yoga (which was a new experience), and I've kept it up on a weekly basis ever since. I also use positive affirmations (short, positive statements repeated regularly to promote positive thinking).

'In a way, work was also part of my "medicine". For a period, I was only able to work from home, but technology and a supportive team meant that I was able to keep my working life as normal as possible, through what was an extremely traumatic experience, not only for me, but for my young family too.

'Work felt like a way of maintaining normality when it felt like my whole life was changing for ever. Working each day was engaging my mind and keeping me mentally active. I was keen and able to work as much as I sensibly could. I know that I am quite motivated by my work because I'm passionate about it and enjoy it, so I asked my HR colleague to be the "angel on my shoulder" whenever it looked like I was trying to take on too much.

'For me, I had to teach my brain to default to a positive thought-cycle. Getting outside and for short walks helped, as did laughter – even just watching a bit of comedy on TV. When I was able to return to the office, my first feelings were ones of relief at being back with people I'd worked alongside for years, as well as a sense of achievement. But at the same time, commuting into the office was a big barrier to getting back into the office environment. My brain had gone into a cycle to tell itself that I couldn't do it, so that was something the CBT helped me break through. CBT paired with exercise therapy was the treatment that got me back to 'life', and other elements – such as mindfulness, meditation, yoga and treating myself well – supported that.'

Gwen, 30

'I had been ill for over six months when I received my diagnosis of ME/CFS. It was having a profound impact on my life at the time – I was unable to work, unable to do any exercise other than short walks, my social life and relationships were compromised, I wasn't able to live independently and look after myself properly, so I moved back in with my parents.

'Once I had my diagnosis of ME/CFS confirmed, I was fortunate enough to be referred to a therapist. I worked with her for eight months, where we created a programme tailored to my recovery. Firstly, we understood my baseline of activity, rest and sleep and sought to increase (for example, exercise or a social event) or decrease (for example, sleep), where appropriate. We also explored my thoughts, feelings and behaviours that were contributing to maintaining the condition, and how to challenge these.

'The process wasn't easy – there were lots of tears, despair and a lot of hard work, but I trusted in the process, and I trusted my specialist. She guided me, challenged me and helped me reframe my condition, focus on progress and what I could do, versus what I couldn't. Exercise, improving sleep quality (rather than quantity), challenging assumptions about what it means to have ME/CFS, and sustainably increasing activity in a controlled way have helped me make a lot of progress with recovery.

'Unfortunately, you don't get a "day off" or a "holiday" from ME/CFS. So following the programme consistently every day was the hardest part. I believe it was also the key to the progress I've made, though, and crucial in avoiding any kind of boom-and-bust, even when I felt so tired that I couldn't put one foot in front of the other.

'I also had a lot of help from family and loved ones, who were there and able to best support me, once I knew how to articulate what I needed from them – in my case, the help I needed from them was that they would help to hold me to account.

'I am now back at work after a phased return over a number of months. I jog three times a week, am back living independently with friends and am living as "normal" a life as possible in a global pandemic. Now I am focusing on keeping the good habits engrained, maintaining boundaries and not panicking if I have a few days where my symptoms are worse.

'I hope my story will bring hope, if you are in a similar situation. I remember well how disheartening the stories on the internet were, when I was looking. I would not have believed I would be in this position a year ago and I want you to know it is possible that things can get better.'

Louise, 37

'It started at the end of 2018. I'd had one of the best years of my life: I'd bought and moved into my own home, run my second marathon and was enjoying volunteering, alongside my career as a civil servant. It felt like things were really taking off for me, but I then fell ill with what we think was the flu, or some kind of virus. I assumed it would be like any other illness and I'd get better and so, after a few days off, I returned to work. However, a week afterwards my mum had to call an ambulance because I just couldn't get out of bed.

'I went to the doctors: my blood tests were clear, as was a brain scan. On paper, I was the picture of health, but in person it was a different story. I felt weak, my throat hurt, my periods stopped, my skin was sore, my mouth was full of ulcers and I would have sensory overload.

'My journey has been three years of trial and error. By the start of 2020 my symptoms had improved to the extent that I was back to working full-time, but then the pandemic hit and I had to shield. I had twelve weeks of not going out: I completely stopped, and my body just lost all its strength again.

'I went back to work for a day, fell over and broke my arm and I went downhill. While I was off from work again, my GP told me that "people with ME don't work". I became quite depressed and was worried I was going to lose my job. Then, sitting with friends one evening, I decided I had to do something, so I made an appointment with a specialist. I also began to research ME/CFS for myself, especially the nervous system, so that I am better informed. For me, this has definitely taken the fear factor away.

'Now I am back at work again full-time, and so far it is going well. I have been able to manage my symptoms and not be as fearful. But that's not to say it is always easy: my role involves being on call during evenings and weekends, and that has been a struggle, because no one week has a set "routine" or body clock, and that is partly why I struggled to get back to where I was. I do still have flare-ups – waking up in the middle of the night feeling feverish and like my glands are swollen.

'Everywhere you look, people tell you this is the new normal for you, and the negative stories are easier to find than the positive, so I decided to set up an Instagram account, called @mindandbody_connected, to link up people at the start of their journey, but also those who have come through the other side.

'I'm fortunate to have a great support network, but sometimes you just want to communicate with people who know, from personal experience, what you are going through – and the account helps with that. If only I had had that network at the start, to connect with people with a positive outlook. I get a lot of private messages from people who just don't know where to start. Everyone's experience of ME/CFS is so different, and I know my approach won't work for everyone, but if I can help just one person through social media, then it is worth it.'

Sue, 59

'I became ill in 2006. My job involved running a small team in a drug and alcohol rehab service and, in retrospect, I can see that I was struggling with fatigue and workplace stress. I fell ill with a chest infection that turned into pneumonia, and I never really recovered from it. My chest-infection symptoms left me, but I was left with the classic symptoms of physical and mental fatigue.

'In the back of my mind I kept thinking, "Is it ME/CFS?" and I kept pushing it away. I said to my doctor at one point, "Whatever you do, don't tell me that's what's wrong with me", but six months after onset I received my diagnosis.

'I was referred to a specialist clinic, and my focus was very much about learning strategies on getting me back to work. I learned pacing, and they helped me plan a staged return to work for a few hours a few mornings a week. I changed to a different role, but although the work was less pressured, I just couldn't cope at all. I felt like I was in a glass cage, and I had to make the decision to retire on medical grounds.

'After retiring, I went downhill mentally. I was depressed, frustrated and angry. I could do anything in my mind when lying down, but in reality I struggled with fatigue, I'd get dizzy and fall over. I'd always had a great social life seeing bands, live music and going out with friends, but that all stopped. I'd go out and after an hour I'd be half asleep at the table, so over time it became easier not to go out.

'I tried acupuncture, healing, hypnotherapy, had every test to rule out other causes. I felt a lot of shame that people might think that if I only tried harder, then I would be okay. I also developed pain and migraines, and in 2012 I ended up being diagnosed with fibromyalgia on top of the ME/CFS and was referred to a pain clinic, and this is where things started changing for the better. The clinic was very into patient involvement, and there were a number of volunteers. I was asked to become a volunteer, and this is the point at which I started getting some hope back. I had skills because of my background, but here was a group of people who knew I was ill, but they believed in me and gave me the opportunity and something to focus on. Very, very gradually I felt that my symptoms were melting.

'The thing I always come back to is the balance between rest and movement and finding out what is right for you. For me, I think that had I physically moved earlier, then the symptoms and the pain might not have got as bad as they did. Another thing I would recommend is really learning how to relax: for me, it is not watching TV or seeing friends, but really slowing down and practising mindfulness and meditation.

'The way I describe it to people is that I felt like a power station at night, except that all but one of the lights had gone out. I was still there, but I wasn't making energy or doing anything worthwhile. Gradually more and more lights are coming on.'

Hannah, 25

'I was on holiday when I was twelve when I first started feeling unwell. I had a virus, and it just didn't get better. I was left with an overriding feeling of weakness and exhaustion, like a flu that never really left me.

'For the first couple of years I was bedbound most of the day. I could manage a short walk to the kitchen and back, but that was about it. I struggled with normal activities and personal care. My whole life was completely changed. I never went back to school. Instead I had "hospital education" with tutors. At the start I could only manage short spells, but it built up to the point where a tutor would come to my house three times a week.

'The first year after being unwell the big aim was finding a diagnosis. It was a long process getting a diagnosis, lots of doctors' appointments. Because the

initial focus was on my physical health and learning to
live with my ME/CFS, I'd almost forgotten that my
teenage years were a time for learning.

'It was a big adjustment not having the normal
interactions you would expect from being at school, like
being with your friends, getting to know your teachers –
all the things you do as a teenager – and I missed out on
that. But when I started learning again, even though it
was exhausting at times, I found I had really missed it.

'I worked with a local ME/CFS team, having
physiotherapy and sessions with an occupational
therapist, and structure was a big thing. I find that even
now I really need structure in my life; even just having
one thing to work towards in a day really helps me.

'After five years with the hospital education team, a
few GCSE grades and my physical health improving,
I went to college. College was a big turning point for
me: my health was improving and I was working
towards vocational qualifications in health and
social care.

'I'm twenty-five now and work four days a week as a
healthcare assistant in a hospice. Even at my lowest point
I always knew I wanted to do something in healthcare.
I had thought it would just be a pipe dream, but I've
achieved what I set out to do.

'In terms of recovery, I do have days where I feel a bit
tired, but overall, physically, I feel very well. The mental
side of recovery has taken longer. I probably get

overwhelmed more easily than the next person. When I was younger I found it difficult to talk about how I felt.

'I do feel proud of myself. You have to take a step back and look at what you have achieved. Don't compare yourself to other people and their experiences. For me, having things to focus on was key. I had to make sure I had tiny things to focus on in the day, to get me through, whether it was watching a bit of a new programme, reading a few pages of a book, seeing a friend or my education.

'And patience was a big thing. It can be hard when you don't know what the future will look like, but have patience and never lose hope.'

Chris, 37

'I was sporty, doing a fairly demanding job with a long commute, in addition to normal life challenges. Then I caught what I thought was a cold (I've since been told it was Epstein–Barr virus). At first I tried to shake it off and carried on working and training for an upcoming triathlon, but I didn't feel quite right.

'About eight weeks after first falling ill I remember being at work and trying to stand up from my chair to go to the bathroom, and I felt absolutely awful. I asked to speak to my boss, and as soon I got in the meeting room I just broke down. My boss sent me home and I agreed to go to the doctor. I genuinely left that meeting thinking I would be back at work the following week, but unfortunately that wasn't the case.

'I went from being one of the fittest people I knew to someone who couldn't walk to the end of their road. The symptoms were varied, but at times it felt like my whole body was inflamed – for example, when I ran my fingers through my hair, it felt like even my hair follicles were inflamed. One of the toughest symptoms was the waves of overwhelming fatigue, where it would take all my physical and mental strength to keep my eyes open.

'I kept getting signed off from work, to the point where I had no idea if I would ever work again, let alone take part in sport. I was calling to cancel races I'd already booked to compete in, in the coming months. This was when I experienced a real turning point. A race organizer called Mark, whom I had never met or spoken to (save for emailing to see if there was a chance of an entry-related refund), offered to call me, because both he and his wife had had ME/CFS. It sounds dramatic, but that phone call saved my life. Even though he didn't know me at all, Mark took the time to speak to me for two hours. He told me how he and his wife had been through ME/CFS, but that they had recovered, and that recovery can be possible.

'I had CBT, but what I enjoyed most about it was talking through things with someone who had experience of helping others who were in a similar situation to me, rather than the therapy itself. For me, the hope that call gave me was a crucial thing. In particular, helping me not to limit my expectations and asking "why not?" as opposed to being afraid to push my boundaries. ME/CFS is such a wide term, and just because therapy works for one person doesn't mean it always works for another.

'At times I struggled to sleep at night, and I feel that resolving this was fundamental. It was very difficult. I fought not to fall asleep when I experienced the waves of fatigue, to give me the best chance of being tired at night. I rationalized that the waves of tiredness were not "genuine" fatigue, but rather my body and mind's attempt to protect me from perceived over-exertion (even when I had done zero activity or movement).

'I also slowly started to exercise, beginning with just walking for five minutes a day. There were times when I would come back and my throat would be inflamed and sore, and I would worry I had pushed myself too far, but I still returned the next day to do the same walk. My recovery and progression were slow, so that my body and mind would become aligned to what my new thresholds were.

'Over time I progressed to longer walks and then eventually to some pretty swift walking! I must have looked silly – people would laugh as they passed me in their cars – but I didn't care; they didn't know my back-story.

'I ended up running five times a week, so that I became fitter than before. Of course I did have setbacks, where I would be really worried and think to myself, "Is this all starting up again?" The symptoms were there, but I was trying not to acknowledge them. It is incredible how, by not acknowledging the symptoms, over time they disappeared. It was as if my normal baseline had been readjusted. If you had told me at the outset that I would be where I am now, I would not have believed it, but it is hope that has done that for me – it gave me the scope to believe.

'If you come through this, you will be stronger than anyone you know.'

Conclusion: Living with ME/CFS

Whether you are worried that your current fatigue symptoms are due to ME/CFS or already have a diagnosis and have completed assessment and treatment or rehabilitation in a specialist ME/CFS centre, we hope the information and advice in this book have given you the clarity and confidence you need to take charge of your own health.

Apart from in children and young adults, the outlook for people with ME/CFS is currently guarded, and while recovery is possible and we have witnessed it, the likelihood of a complete remission or cure is, sadly, currently quite low. But maintaining hope is absolutely vital, and the best chance of minimizing any adverse impact on your life comes when healthcare professionals are engaged early, specialist advice is provided promptly and support is offered to keep people engaged in education or employment where appropriate, with modifications where necessary.

We believe there are some key messages to take away from this book:

- **Don't delay seeking help and advice:** If severe fatigue is affecting your everyday life, please see a healthcare professional. Do not wait until your symptoms become unbearable.

- **Remember that good care is not just about diagnostics and medication**: Consider your overall health and well-being and make use of the advice we have provided on diet and self-management. We have provided links to apps and techniques for improving sleep and stress management (see Further Reading and Resources on page 225), which we believe are important as part of a holistic approach to living with ME/CFS. Make sure you take time out to do things that you enjoy and boost your self-esteem.

- **Talk about your experiences with others**: Slowly but surely, society is getting better at talking openly about ME/CFS. Well-known figures – including the round-the-world yachtswoman Clare Francis and the director of the 1981 film *Chariots of Fire*, David Puttnam – have spoken candidly about their experience of ME/CFS. Lord Puttnam is a patron and Clare Francis the president of the charity Action for ME, and for us they are inspiring examples of people who continue to have fulfilling careers that enrich the lives of others, despite living with ME/CFS. We can all play a part in raising awareness of ME/CFS, be it in the workplace, among friends or around the dinner table.

- **Keep an eye out for developments in our understanding of ME/CFS**: The next few years will see an explosion of papers published specifically relating to post-viral fatigue. While these are exciting times, it is likely that there will be many false dawns before we reach the sunlight uplands that so many hope for. Chapter 5 set out the high bar to be achieved before it can safely be concluded that a proposed disease mechanism is established or that a novel treatment is better than a placebo, and far too many advocates in the past have gone from the results of laboratory investigation to treatment recommendations without the crucial step of randomized controlled trials to test their hypothesis. While we are all impatient for novel therapeutics, proving effectiveness is vital before alterations to treatment guidelines can sensibly be made.

- **Never give up hope:** While we believe it is important to be realistic about the likelihood of complete cure, it is also far easier to find examples online of people who are severely affected than of the many who have recovered, or who live well despite ongoing ME/CFS. We have tried to redress the balance a little in this book, by sharing some real-life examples of people with even the most severe forms of the condition who have managed to get their lives and careers back on track. While not in any way wishing to disrespect or detract from the poor experiences of those who are severely affected, through no fault of their own, and who need society's advocacy and support (and of course better therapeutics), we believe it is vital that recovery stories are believed, understood, learned from and, most importantly, not undermined.

Notes

Introduction

1 L. Bateman, A. C. Bested, H. F. Bonilla et al. (2021), 'Myalgic Encephalomyelitis/Chronic Fatigue Syndrome: Essentials of Diagnosis and Management', *Mayo Clinic Proceedings*, 96 (11), pp.2861–78, doi.org/10.1016/j.mayocp.2021.07.004

2 M. van't Leven, G. A. Zielhuis, J. W. van der Meer et al. (2010), 'Fatigue and chronic fatigue syndrome-like complaints in the general population', *European Journal of Public Health*, 20 (3), pp.251–7, doi.org/10.1093/eurpub/ckp113

3 W. Wojcik, D. Armstrong and R. Kanaan (2011), 'Chronic fatigue syndrome: Labels, meanings and consequences', *Journal of Psychosomatic Research*, 70 (6), pp.500–4, doi.org/10.1016/j.jpsychores.2011.02.002

4 Committee on the Diagnostic Criteria for Myalgic Encephalomyelitis/Chronic Fatigue Syndrome et al. (2015), 'Beyond Myalgic Encephalomyelitis/Chronic Fatigue Syndrome: Redefining an Illness', *National Academies*, doi.org/10.17226/19012

5 S. Wessely (1995), 'The epidemiology of chronic fatigue syndrome', *Epidemiologic Reviews*, 17 (1), pp.139–51, doi.org/10.1093/oxfordjournals.epirev.a036170

6 L. A. Jason et al. (1999), 'A community-based study of chronic fatigue syndrome', *Archives of Internal Medicine*, 159 (18), pp.2129–37, doi.org/10.1001/archinte.159.18.2129

7 National Institute for Health and Care Excellence/NICE (2007), 'Chronic fatigue syndrome/myalgic encephalomyelitis (or encephalopathy): Diagnosis and management', www.nice.org.uk/guidance/cg53

8 Bateman et al. (2021), 'Myalgic Encephalomyelitis/Chronic Fatigue Syndrome: Essentials of Diagnosis and Management', doi.org/10.1016/j.mayocp.2021.07.004

9 E. Roberts et al. (2016), 'Mortality of people with chronic fatigue syndrome: A retrospective cohort study in England and Wales from the South London and Maudsley NHS Foundation Trust Biomedical Research Centre (SLaM BRC) Clinical Record Interactive Search (CRIS) Register', *The Lancet*, 387 (10028), pp.1638–43, doi.org/10.1016/S0140-6736(15)01223-4

10 L. Chu et al. (2021), 'Identifying and managing suicidality in myalgic encephalomyelitis/chronic fatigue syndrome', *Healthcare*, 9 (6), doi.org/10.3390/healthcare9060629

11 Y. Nakatomi et al. (2014), 'Neuroinflammation in Patients with Chronic Fatigue Syndrome/Myalgic Encephalomyelitis: An ^{11}C-(R)-PK11195 PET Study', *Journal of Nuclear Medicine*, 55 (6), pp.945–50, doi.org/10.2967/jnumed.113.131045

12 M. B. VanElzakker et al. (2019), 'Neuroinflammation and Cytokines in Myalgic Encephalomyelitis/Chronic Fatigue Syndrome (ME/CFS): A Critical Review of Research Methods', *Frontiers in Neurology*, 9 (1033), doi.org/10.3389/fneur.2018.01033

1. Classical ME/CFS

1 E. M. Lacerda et al. (2019), 'A logistic regression analysis of risk factors in ME/CFS pathogenesis', *BMC Neurology*, 19 (1), doi.org/10.1186/s12883-019-1468-2

2 F. Albright, K. Light, A. Light et al. (2011), 'Evidence for a heritable predisposition to chronic fatigue syndrome', *BMC Neurology*, 11 (62), doi.org/10.1186/1471-2377-11-62

3 K. Kato et al. (2006), 'Premorbid predictors of chronic fatigue', *Archives of General Psychiatry*, 63 (11), pp.1267–72, doi.org/10.1001/archpsyc.63.11.1267

4 Ibid.

5 J. A. Leonard et al. (2021), 'Risks for developing myalgic encephalomyelitis/chronic fatigue syndrome in college students following infectious mononucleosis: A prospective cohort study', *Clinical Infectious Diseases: An Official Publication of the Infectious Diseases Society of America*, 73 (11), e3740–e3746, doi.org/10.1093/cid/ciaa1886

6 M. Maes, E. Bosmans, E. Suy et al. (1991), 'A further exploration of the relationships between immune parameters and the HPA-axis activity in depressed patients', *Psychological Medicine*, 21 (2), pp.313–20, doi.org/10.1017/s0033291700020419

7 A. L. Komaroff and D. S. Buchwald (1998), 'Chronic fatigue syndrome: An update', *Annual Review of Medicine*, 49, pp.1–13, doi.org/10.1146/annurev.med.49.1.1

8 J. Daniels et al. (2017), 'Anxiety and depression in chronic fatigue syndrome/myalgic encephalomyelitis (CFS/ME): Examining the incidence of health anxiety in CFS/ME', *Psychology and Psychotherapy*, 90 (3), pp.502–9, doi.org/10.1111/papt.12118

9 A. Berende, J. M. Hadewych et al. (2016), 'Randomised trial of longer term therapy for symptoms attributed to Lyme disease', *The New England Journal of Medicine*, 374 (13), pp. 1209–20, doi.org/10.1056/NEJMoa1505425

10 ME/CFS Independent Working Group (2002), 'A report of the CFS/ME working group: Report to the chief medical officer of an independent working group', www.meassociation.org.uk/wp-content/uploads/CMO-Report-2002.pdf

11 T. Norris et al. (2017), 'Natural course of chronic fatigue syndrome/myalgic encephalomyelitis in adolescents', *Archives of Disease in Childhood*, 102 (6), pp.522–8, doi.org/10.archdischild-2016-311198

12 E. Crawley, S. M. Collin, P. D. White et al. (2013), 'Treatment outcome in adults with chronic fatigue syndrome: A prospective study in England based on the CFS/ME National Outcomes Database', *QJM: Monthly Journal of the Association of Physicians*, 106 (6), pp.555–65, doi.org/10.1093/qjmed/hct061

13 S. M. Collin and E. Crawley (2017), 'Specialist treatment of chronic fatigue syndrome/ME: A cohort study among adult patients in England', *BMC Health Service Research*, 17 (1), doi.org/10.1186/s12913-017-2437-3

14 Centers for Disease Control & Prevention (2021), 'Chronic Fatigue Syndrome: Basic facts', www.cdc.gov/cfs/cfsbasicfacts.html

2. PVFS and Other Fatigue-Related Syndromes

1 Ehlers–Danlos Society, 'The Beighton Score: How to Assess Joint Hypermobility', ehlers-danlos.com/wp-content/uploads/Beighton-Score-2017.pdf

2 A. J. Hakim et al. (2004), 'The genetic epidemiology of joint hypermobility: A population study of female twins', *Arthritis and Rheumatism*, 50 (8), pp.2640–4, doi.org/10.1002/art.20376

3 A. Hakim and G. Rodney (2003), 'Joint hypermobility', *Best Practice and Research: Clinical Rheumatology*, 17 (6), pp.989–1004, doi.org/10.1016/j.berh.2003.08.001

4 Hakim et al. (2004), 'The genetic epidemiology of joint hypermobility', doi.org/10.1002/art.20376

5 F. Malfait et al. (2017), 'The 2017 international classification of the Ehlers–Danlos syndromes', *American Journal of Medical Genetics*, 175 (1), pp.8–26, doi.org/10.1002/ajmg.c.31552

6 A. J. Hakim et al. (2017), 'Chronic fatigue in Ehlers–Danlos syndrome-hypermobile type', *American Journal of Medical Genetics*, 175 (1), pp.175–80, doi.org/10.1002/ajmg.c.31542

7 J. A. Eccles et al. (2021), 'Beyond bones: The relevance of variants of connective tissue (hypermobility) to fibromyalgia, ME/CFS and controversies surrounding diagnostic classification: An observational study', *Clinical Medicine*, 21 (1), pp.53–8, doi.org/10.7861/clinmed.2020-0743

8 Ehlers–Danlos Society, 'Hypermobile Ehlers–Danlos Syndrome: Clinical Description and Natural History', www.ehlers-danlos.com/2017-eds-classification-non-experts/hypermobile-ehlers-danlos-syndrome-clinical-description-natural-history/

9 A. Bulbena et al. (2017), 'Psychiatric and psychological aspects in the Ehlers–Danlos syndromes', *American Journal of Medical Genetics*, 175 (1), pp.237–45, doi.org/10.1002/ajmg.c.31544

10 NHS.uk, 'Fibromyalgia: Overview' (2019), www.nhs.uk/conditions/fibromyalgia/

11 NICE (2021), 'Chronic pain (primary and secondary) in over 16s: Assessment of all chronic pain and management of chronic primary pain', www.nice.org.uk/guidance/ng193

12 R. S. Sheldon et al. (2015), '2015 Heart Rhythm Society Expert Consensus Statement on the Diagnosis and Treatment of Postural Tachycardia Syndrome, Inappropriate Sinus Tachycardia, and Vasovagal Syncope', *Heart Rhythm*, 12 (6), e41–63, doi.org/10.1016/j.hrthm.2015.03.029

13 I. Lewis et al. (2013), 'Clinical characteristics of a novel subgroup of chronic fatigue syndrome patients with postural orthostatic tachycardia syndrome', *Journal of Internal Medicine*, 273 (5), pp.501–10, doi.org/10.1111/joim.12022

14 A. J. Miller et al. (2020), 'Prevalence of hypermobile Ehlers–Danlos syndrome in postural orthostatic tachycardia syndrome', *Autonomic Neuroscience: Basic & Clinical*, doi.org/10.1016/j.autneu.2020.102637

15 Q. Fu et al. (2010), 'Cardiac origins of the postural orthostatic tachycardia syndrome', *Journal of the American College of Cardiology*, 55 (25), pp.2858–68, doi.org/10.1016/j.jacc.2010.02.043

16 S. Masuki et al. (2007), 'Excessive heart rate response to orthostatic stress in postural tachycardia syndrome is not caused by anxiety', *Journal of Applied Physiology*, 102 (3), pp.896–903, doi.org/10.1152/japplphysiol.00927.2006

17 Sheldon et al. (2015), '2015 Heart Rhythm Society Expert Consensus Statement', doi.org/10.1016/j.hrthm.2015.03.029

18 R. Winker et al. (2005), 'Endurance exercise training in orthostatic intolerance: A randomized, controlled trial',

Hypertension, 45 (3), pp.391–8, doi.org/10.1161/01.HYP.0000156540.25707.af

19 A. Kohn and C. Chang (2020), 'The Relationship between Hypermobile Ehlers–Danlos Syndrome (hEDS), postural orthostatic tachycardia syndrome (POTS), and mast cell activation syndrome (MCAS)', *Clinical Reviews in Allergy and Immunology*, 58 (3), pp.273–97, doi.org/10.1007/s12016-019-08755-8

20 C. R. Weiler et al. (2019), 'AAAAI Mast Cell Disorders Committee Work Group Report: Mast cell activation syndrome (MCAS) diagnosis and management', *The Journal of Allergy and Clinical Immunology*, 144 (4), pp.883–96, doi.org/10.1016/j.jaci.2019.08.023

3. Theories Regarding Causation

1 V. C. Lombardi et al. (2009), 'Detection of an infectious retrovirus, XMRV, in blood cells of patients with chronic fatigue syndrome', *Science*, 326 (5952), pp.585–9, doi.org/10.1126/science.1179052

2 B. Alberts (2011), 'Retraction', *Science*, 334 (6063), p.1636, doi.org/10.1126/science.334.6063.1636-a

3 P. M. Visscher et al. (2017), '10 years of GWAS discovery: Biology, function, and translation', *American Journal of Human Genetics*, 101 (1), pp.5–22, doi.org/10.1016/j.ajhg.2017.06.005

4 K. Bjornevik, M. Cortese et al. (2022), 'Longitudinal analysis reveals high prevalence of Epstein–Barr virus associated with multiple sclerosis', *Science*, 375 (6578), pp.296–301

5 A. Berende et al. (2016), 'Randomized Trial of Longer-Term Therapy for Symptoms Attributed to Lyme Disease', *The New England Journal of Medicine*, 374 (13), pp.1209–20, doi.org/10.1056/NEJMoa1505425

6 S. P. Keijmel et al. (2017), 'Effectiveness of Long-Term Doxycycline Treatment and Cognitive-Behavioral Therapy on Fatigue Severity in Patients with Q Fever Fatigue Syndrome (Qure Study): A Randomized Controlled Trial', *Clinical Infectious Diseases*, 64 (8), pp.998–1005, doi.org/10.1093/cid/cix013

7 Z. Kmietowicz (2010), 'Wakefield is struck off for the "serious and wide-ranging findings against him"', *British Medical Journal,* doi.org/10.1136/bmj.c2803

8 The Editors of *The Lancet* (2010), 'Retraction – Ileal-lymphoid-nodular hyperplasia, non-specific colitis, and pervasive developmental disorder in children', *The Lancet*, 375 (9713), p.445, doi.org/10.1016/S0140-6736(10)60175-4

9 C. Tomas and J. Newton (2018), 'Metabolic abnormalities in chronic fatigue syndrome/myalgic encephalomyelitis: A mini-review', *Biochemical Society Transactions*, 46 (3), pp.547–53, doi.org/10.1042/BST20170503

10 C. Tomas et al. (2019), 'Assessing cellular energy dysfunction in CFS/ME using a commercially available laboratory test', *Scientific Reports*, 9 (1), doi.org/10.1038/s41598-019-47966-z

11 D. L. Arnold et al. (1984), 'Excessive intracellular acidosis of skeletal muscle on exercise in a patient with a post-viral exhaustion/fatigue syndrome: A 31P nuclear magnetic resonance study', *The Lancet*, 1 (8391), pp.1367–9, doi.org/10.1016/s0140-6736(84)91871-3

12 Tomas and Newton (2018), 'Metabolic abnormalities in chronic fatigue syndrome/myalgic encephalomyelitis', doi. org/10.1042/BST20170503

13 R. McKenzie, A. O'Fallon, J. Dale, M. Demitrack et al. (1998), 'Low-dose hydrocortisone for treatment of chronic fatigue syndrome: A randomized controlled trial', *Journal of the American Medical Association*, 280 (12), pp.1061–6, doi.org/ 10.1001/jama.280.12.1061

14 A. J. Cleare, E. Heap, G. S. Malhi et al. (1999), 'Low-dose hydrocortisone in chronic fatigue syndrome: A randomised crossover trial', *The Lancet*, 353 (9151), pp.455–8, doi:10.1016/ S0140-6736(98)04074-4

15 A. J. Cleare, A. Roberts, A. Papadopoulos et al. (2004), 'Cognitive behavioural therapy normalises HPA axis dysfunction in chronic fatigue syndrome', *European Neuropsychopharmacology*, 14 (3), p.389, doi.org/10.1016/S0924-977X(04)80581-9

16 M. Hotopf, N. Noah and S. Wessely (1996), 'Chronic fatigue and minor psychiatric morbidity after viral meningitis: A controlled study', *Journal of Neurology, Neurosurgery and Psychiatry*, 60 (5), pp.504–9, doi.org/10.1136/jnnp.60.5.504

17 M. D. Mitchell, P. Gehrman, M. Perlis et al. (2012), 'Comparative effectiveness of cognitive behavioral therapy for insomnia: A systematic review', *BMC Family Practice*, 13 (40), doi.org/10.1186/1471-2296-13-40

18 E. Roberts et al. (2016), 'Mortality of people with chronic fatigue syndrome: A retrospective cohort study in England and Wales from the South London and Maudsley NHS Foundation Trust Biomedical Research Centre (SLaM BRC) Clinical Record Interactive Search (CRIS) Register',

The Lancet, 387 (10028), pp.1638–43, doi.org/10.1016/S0140-6736(15)01223-4

19 NICE (2020), 'Low back pain and sciatica in over 16s: Assessment and management', www.nice.org.uk/guidance/ng59

20 NICE (2021), 'Chronic pain (primary and secondary) in over 16s: Assessment of all chronic pain and management of chronic primary pain', www.nice.org.uk/guidance/ng193

21 NICE (2021), 'Myalgic encephalomyelitis (or encephalopathy)/chronic fatigue syndrome: Diagnosis and management', www.nice.org.uk/guidance/ng206

4. Self-Management Strategies

1 App Annie (2021), 'Pumped up: Health and fitness app downloads rose 30% in a landmark year for mobile wellness', www.appannie.com/en/insights/market-data/health-fitness-downloads-rose-30-percent/

5. Treatment Options: Medications and Supplements

1 R. Sihvonen et al. (2013), 'Arthroscopic partial meniscectomy versus sham surgery for a degenerative meniscal tear', *The New England Journal of Medicine*, 369 (26), pp.2515–24, doi.org/10.1056/NEJMoa1305189

2 ME Action (2019), 'A Letter from Jennifer Brea about Her ME Remission', www.meaction.net/2019/05/21/a-letter-from-jennifer-brea-about-her-me-remission

3 ME Association,meassociation.org.uk/wp-content/uploads/ Forward-ME-Position-Statement-Spinal-Surgery-and-ME-15.10.20.pdf

4 Ø. Fluge et al. (2016), 'Metabolic profiling indicates impaired pyruvate dehydrogenase function in myalgic encephalopathy/chronic fatigue syndrome', *JCI Insight*, 1 (21), e89376, doi. org/10.1172/jci.insight.89376

5 P. K. Peterson et al. (1990), 'A controlled trial of intravenous immunoglobulin G in chronic fatigue syndrome', *The American Journal of Medicine*, 89 (5), pp.554–60, doi.org/10.1016/0002-9343(90)90172-a

6 D. R. Strayer et al. (2012), 'A double-blind, placebo-controlled, randomized, clinical trial of the TLR-3 agonist rintatolimod in severe cases of chronic fatigue syndrome', *PloS One*, 7 (3), e31334, doi.ORG/10.1371/journal.pone.0031334

7 M. E. Roerink et al. (2017), 'Cytokine Inhibition in Patients With Chronic Fatigue Syndrome: A Randomized Trial', *Annals of Internal Medicine*, 166 (8), pp.557–64, doi.org/10.7326/M16-2391

8 R. K. Morriss et al. (2002), 'Neuropsychological performance and noradrenaline function in chronic fatigue syndrome under conditions of high arousal', *Journal of Psychopharmacology*, 163 (2), pp.166–73, doi.org/10.1007/s00213-002-1129-8

9 D. C. Randall et al. (2005), 'Chronic treatment with modafinil may not be beneficial in patients with chronic fatigue syndrome', *Journal of Psychopharmacology*, 19 (6), pp.647–60, doi. org/10.1177/0269881105056531

10 D. Blockmans et al. (2006), 'Does methylphenidate reduce the symptoms of chronic fatigue syndrome?', *The*

American Journal of Medicine, 119 (2), doi.org/10.1016/j.amjmed.2005.07.047

11 G. Montoya et al. (2018), 'KPAX002 as a treatment for Myalgic Encephalomyelitis/Chronic Fatigue Syndrome (ME/CFS): A prospective, randomized trial', *International Journal of Clinical and Experimental Medicine*, 11 (3), pp.2890–900

12 L. G. Olson et al. (2003), 'A pilot randomized controlled trial of dexamphetamine in patients with chronic fatigue syndrome', *Psychosomatics*, 44 (1), pp.38–43, doi.org/10.1176/appi.psy.44.1.38

13 J. L. Young (2013), 'Use of lisdexamfetamine dimesylate in treatment of executive functioning deficits and chronic fatigue syndrome: A double blind, placebo-controlled study', *Psychiatry Research*, 207 (1–2), pp.127–33, doi.org/10.1016/j.psychres.2012.09.007

14 J. G. Montoya et al. (2013), 'Randomized clinical trial to evaluate the efficacy and safety of valganciclovir in a subset of patients with chronic fatigue syndrome', *Journal of Medical Virology*, 85 (12), pp.2101–9, doi.org/10.1002/jmv.23713

15 P. Steinberg et al. (1996), 'Double-blind placebo-controlled study of the efficacy of oral terfenadine in the treatment of chronic fatigue syndrome', *The Journal of Allergy and Clinical Immunology*, 97 (1), pp.119–26, doi.org/10.1016/s0091-6749(96)70290-7

16 M. Maes et al. (2009), 'Coenzyme Q10 deficiency in myalgic encephalomyelitis/chronic fatigue syndrome (ME/CFS) is related to fatigue, autonomic and neurocognitive symptoms and is another risk factor explaining the early mortality in ME/CFS due to cardiovascular disorder', *Neuro Endocrinology Letters*, 30 (4), pp.470–6

17 M. M. Peel et al. (2005), 'A randomized controlled trial of coenzyme Q10 for fatigue in the late-onset sequelae of poliomyelitis', *Complementary Therapies in Medicine*, 23 (6), pp. 789–93, doi.org/10.1016/j.ctim.2015.09.002

18 L. C. Heap et al. (1999), 'Vitamin B status in patients with chronic fatigue syndrome', *Journal of the Royal Society of Medicine*, 92 (4), pp.183–5, doi.org/10.1177/014107689909200405

19 A. Caso Marasco et al. (1999), 'Double-blind study of a multivitamin complex supplemented with ginseng extract', *Drugs under Experimental and Clinical Research*, 22 (6), pp.323–9

20 J. E. Kaslow et al. (1989), 'Liver extract-folic acid-cyanocobalamin vs placebo for chronic fatigue syndrome', *Archives of Internal Medicine*, 149 (11), pp.2501–3

21 I. M. Cox et al. (1991), 'Red blood cell magnesium and chronic fatigue syndrome', *The Lancet*, 337 (8744), pp.757–60, doi.org/10.1016/0140-6736(91)91371-z

22 NICE (2021), 'Chronic pain (primary and secondary) in over 16s: Assessment of all chronic pain and management of chronic primary pain', www.nice.org.uk/guidance/ng193

6. Nutrition and Food

1 J. M. Yano (2015), 'Indigenous bacteria from the gut microbiota regulate host serotonin biosynthesis', *Cell*, 161 (2), pp.264–76, doi.org/10.1016/j.cell.2015.02.047

2 Public Health England (2016), 'Government dietary recommendations: Government recommendations for energy and nutrients for males and females aged 1–18 years and 19+ years', assets.publishing.service.gov.uk/government/

uploads/system/uploads/attachment_data/file/618167/government_dietary_recommendations.pdf

3 NICE (2021), 'Myalgic encephalomyelitis (or encephalopathy)/chronic fatigue syndrome: Diagnosis and management', www.nice.org.uk/guidance/ng206

7. ME/CFS, Work and Education

1 G. Waddell and K. Burton (2006), 'Is work good for your health and well-being?', assets.publishing.service.gov.uk/government/uploads/system/uploads/attachment_data/file/214326/hwwb-is-work-good-for-you.pdf

2 Department for Work and Pensions (2006), 'Is work good for your health and well-being? An independent review', www.gov.uk/government/publications/is-work-good-for-your-health-and-well-being

3 Equality Act (2010), www.legislation.gov.uk/ukpga/2010/15/contents

4 NICE (2019), 'Workplace health: long-term sickness absence and capability to work', www.nice.org.uk/guidance/ng146

9. Questions to Ask Your Healthcare Professional

1 NHS Digital (2021), 'Appointments in General Practice – September 2021', www.digital.nhs.uk/data-and-information/publications/statistical/appointments-in-general-practice/september-2021

Further Reading and Resources

ME/CFS professional organizations and charities

UK

Action for ME, UK charity, www.actionforme.org.uk
British Association for ME/CFS (BACME), a multidisciplinary organization for UK professionals caring for patients with ME/CFS, www.bacme.info
ME Association, UK charity, www.meassociation.org.uk
Tymes Trust, a charity dedicated to children and young people with ME/CFS and their families, www.tymestrust.org

Worldwide

American ME and CFS Society, a non-profit organization focused on patient needs, including a doctor and clinic database, www.ammes.org
Association Française du Syndrome de Fatigue Chronique et de Fibromyalgie, French patient-run support organization, www.asso-sfc.org
Associated New Zealand ME Society (ANZMES), support and advice site, www.anzmes.org.nz

European ME Alliance, a group of organizations involved in supporting patients with ME/CFS, www.euro-me.org

Fatigatio e.V., German patient organization, www.fatigatio.de

International Association for CFS/ME (IACFS/ME), a global non-profit group aimed at professionals, www.iacfsme.org

Irish ME/CFS Association, a volunteer-run organization, irishmecfs.org/contact.html

Irish ME Trust, information and counselling service, www.imet.ie/index.html

Japan ME Association, a non-profit organization advocating for patients, www.mecfsjapan.com

ME Association, Danish non-profit organization, www.me-foreningen.dk

ME/CFS Australia, charity, www.mecfs.org.au

ME/CFS Foundation Netherlands, patient organization, www.mecvs.nl

ME/CFS Foundation South Africa, www.mecfssa.org

National ME/FM Action Network, Canadian charity dedicated to ME/FS and fibromyalgia, www.mefmaction.com

Solve ME/CFS, USA-based non-profit organization, www.solvecfs.org

Guidelines

National Institute for Health and Care Excellence (NICE), 'Myalgic encephalomyelitis (or encephalopathy)/chronic fatigue syndrome: diagnosis and management', www.nice.org.uk/guidance/ng206

Health and well-being apps

Calm, meditation app, www.calm.com
Headspace, guided meditation app, www.headspace.com
Insight Timer, guided meditation app, www.insighttimer.com
Sleepio, evidence-based six-week sleep programme, www.
 sleepio.com

Sleep resources

Sleep Foundation, medically reviewed sleep-health information, www.sleepfoundation.org
sleepOT, information and networking site for occupational
 therapists interested in sleep, www.sleepot.org

Nutrition

British Association for Parenteral and Enteral Nutrition
 (BAPEN), self-screening malnutrition tool, www.bapen.org.
 uk/screening-and-must/malnutrition-self-screening-tool
British Dietetic Association (BDA), advice on food and ME/
 CFS, www.bda.uk.com/resource/chronic-fatigue-syndrome-
 diet.html
BDA, advice on food and IBS, www.bda.uk.com/resource/
 irritable-bowel-syndrome-diet.html
BDA, factsheet on malnutrition, www.bda.uk.com/resource/
 malnutrition.html

BDA Freelance Dietitians Specialist Group, database of UK-registered dietitians, www.freelancedietitians.org

IBS Network, charity, www.theibsnetwork.org/diet/

Vegan Society, charity, www.vegansociety.com

Vegan Society, advice on nutrition and health, www.vegansociety.com/resources/nutrition-and-health

Workplace help and support

Access to Work scheme, funding and advice to help you get or stay in work if you have a physical or mental-health condition or disability, www.gov.uk/access-to-work

Advisory, Conciliation and Arbitration Service (ACAS), UK organization offering free advice on employment rights, rules and best practice, www.acas.org.uk

Equality Act 2010, www.legislation.gov.uk/ukpga/2010/15/section/20

Education help and support

Action for ME, support for school, www.actionforme.org.uk/18-and-under/your-education/school/

Action for ME, charity, factsheet on ME/CFS and higher education, www.actionforme.org.uk/support-others/for-teachers-and-schools/higher-and-further-education/

Disabled Students' Allowance, UK-government means-tested support, www.gov.uk/disabled-students-allowance-dsa

Health Conditions in Schools Alliance, a group of charities, healthcare professionals and trade unions that work to ensure children with health conditions get the care they need in school, www.medicalconditionsatschool.org.uk

Special Educational Needs and Disabilities Information Advice and Support Services, information for parents and carers of children and young people with special educational needs and disabilities, www.kids.org.uk/sendiass

Well-known figures with ME/CFS

Clare Francis, author and yachtswoman, www.clarefrancis.com/biography

Lord David Puttnam, director, www.davidputtnam.com

Additional resources

DecodeME, ME/CFS study, www.decodeme.org.uk

C. Tomas and J. Newton (2018), 'Metabolic abnormalities in chronic fatigue syndrome/myalgic encephalomyelitis: A mini-review', *Biochemical Society Transactions*, 46 (3), pp.547–53, doi.org/10.1042/BST20170503

Acknowledgements

Gerald Coakley

To most rheumatologists, people with ME/CFS are not considered to fall within their remit. My interest came from a chance encounter with my friend and colleague Dr Selwyn Richards at an American College of Rheumatology meeting in Boston in 1999. Selwyn had been researching treatments for fibromyalgia, which led to an interest in fatigue, and he is now Clinical Lead for the Dorset ME/CFS service. He advised me that I might find the condition interesting, and he was right.

I learned so much from working with Dr Maurice Lipsedge and with Dr Dinshaw Master, both now retired, but both of whom encouraged me, tactfully suggested some alterations to my naïve early consultation style, and taught me the utility of analogies, reflection and praise in the clinical conversation. Latterly I have been grateful for the support and wisdom of Dr Alastair Santhouse. I am grateful to all three, as well as to Professor Melvyn Lobo and Professor Guy Leschziner, for their helpful comments on earlier versions of this manuscript.

In so far as my patients with ME/CFS have benefited from seeking my opinion (and, sadly, not all have), a major part of their improvement or recovery is due to the diligent and effective treatment of my colleague Gabriella Airey, as well as the team at www.vitality360.co.uk.

I am grateful to the team at Penguin for their patient efforts to get me to meet deadlines and to improve the structure of my jottings, especially Kat Keogh, Lydia Yadi and Susannah Bennett.

Finally, I acknowledge my patients with ME/CFS. I can only admire your fortitude and resilience in the face of a condition that is generally poorly understood, little recognized or researched and often not well supported by healthcare professionals, HR departments, benefits agencies or healthcare insurers. For those who recovered, I celebrate your good fortune and thank you for your trust in me and my team at a difficult time in your life. Our interaction was but brief, and the hard work of recovery all yours. For those who did not recover, I apologize that I could not do more, and I hope that the future will bring new insights and treatments to help you. Where there's life, there is hope.

Beverly Knops

During the last twenty-five years I have worked in three very special multidisciplinary teams: the Bristol Chronic Pain and Fatigue team, Bath Paediatric CFS/ME Service and Vitality360. My thanks go to every single individual in these teams for generously sharing their knowledge and skills with me.

I would like to specifically thank some colleagues and

friends who have supported chapters in this book: diet – Sue Luscombe; work – Amanda Mason and Fiona McKechnie; rehabilitation – Sue Watkins and Liz Dawe. Thank you, I wouldn't have finished on time without you.

I am also grateful to Kat Keogh, who made sense of my ramblings and kept Gerald and me on track.

But most of all I want to acknowledge each and every one of the people with ME/CFS that I have worked with. Your lived experience matters and has contributed hugely to the knowledge that I have shared – and continue to share – with others. Thank you for letting me into your lives.

PREPARING FOR THE PERIMENOPAUSE AND MENOPAUSE

DR LOUISE NEWSON

The *Sunday Times* Number One Bestseller.

Part of the Penguin Life Experts series.

Dr Louise Newson is the UK's leading menopause specialist, and she's determined to help women thrive during the menopause.

Despite being something that almost every woman will experience at some point in their lives, menopause is frequently misdiagnosed and misinformation and stigma are commonplace. Dr Newson demystifies the menopause and explains why every woman should be perimenopause-aware, regardless of their age.

Using new research, expert advice and empowering patient stories from a diverse range of women who have struggled to secure adequate treatment and correct diagnosis, Dr Newson equips readers with expert advice and practical tips. She empowers women to confidently take charge of their health and their changing bodies.

It's never too early to learn about the perimenopause or menopause and this compact guide will provide you with everything you need to know.